Awareness Through Movement® Lessons

The Use of the Eyes in Movement

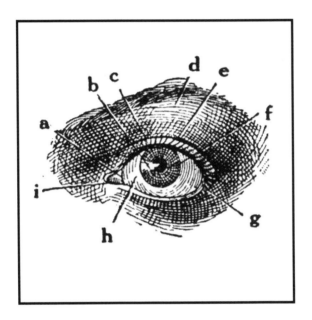

JACK HEGGIE

FELDENKRAIS® RESOURCES

ISBN: 978-0-615-55923-0

Feldenkrais Method®, *Functional Integration®*, *Awareness Through Movement®*, and *Guild Certified Feldenkrais Practitioner®* are service marks of the *Feldenkrais* GUILD® of North America.

Feldenkrais Resources
3680 6th Avenue
San Diego, CA 92103
www.feldenkraisresources.com

Contents

Forward

The book you have before you is slim but packed with little gems. Jack Heggie was a multitalented individual who started out as an engineer and ended up practicing the *Feldenkrais Method*® of Somatic Education. He worked in private practice for decades with people of all ages and with a large variety of requests and complaints. Out of this experience and his extensive reading, Jack created the experiments and exercises in this book. The reader with knowledge of the Bates Method will notice that Jack also drew on the this method, taking some of the Bates exercises and giving them a *Feldenkrais*® flavor. Jack initially was interested in improving his own eyesight, but over time he realized what an essential role the improvement of the eyes could play in a whole host of troubling conditions. If you follow the progression of the experiments and exercises in this book as Jack suggests, you may be surprised to find that the improvement in the functioning of your eyes has affected you positively in other areas as well.

Jack Heggie grew up in Dallas, the son of an airline pilot and a homemaker. Always interested in how things worked, he studied engineering and gained his degree in 1967. Jack worked on various engineering projects into the '70s but found the corporate world stifling and kept changing jobs and locations. After a decade of this, he followed a lifelong dream and set out to sail around the world with a friend (they made it only part way). On his return he took a job on a ship doing early GPS work mapping the bottom of the ocean. This job required that he spend months out at sea. Jack packed a motorcycle on the boat and whenever they came to port he would take off to explore the new terrain. His brother, Jim Heggie, wrote me the following story: "There is one incident many years ago that, to me, has always captured the essence of who my brother was. Just before he left for his defense contract job in the Atlantic, I asked him if he knew where the ship was going. He replied with his characteristic shrug that he didn't know. When I asked, somewhat incredulously, if he didn't care, he replied, "It's not that I don't care, but there are more places that I haven't been than I have, so most anyplace will do.""

The work on the ship left Jack with plenty of free time, and he was always accompanied by stacks of books. During this period he encountered the work of Moshe Feldenkrais who was to provide the key for Jack to bring together his engineering background, his restless intellect and his desire to find work that was more personally meaningful. Moshe Feldenkrais was a pioneer in the field of somatics who applied his background in physics, engineering and martial arts to turn the medical model on its head. Feldenkrais applied an educational learning based approach to many of the pains and neuromuscular problems that commonly plague 20th-century humans with impressive results. The Method was a perfect fit for Jack as he loved to figure things out and what is more challenging than the myriad of ways that humans limit themselves?

Jack visited Feldenkrais in Tel Aviv, where he was living and eventually completed a four-year training to become a *Feldenkrais* practitioner. He became a widely respected teacher of the Method and was known for the effectiveness of his work. He maintained private practice in Boulder, Colorado, where he lived at the end of his life, and in Dallas where he was born. He was particularly critical of the medical profession and had countless stories of clients of who had tried everything and gained relief with Jack's inquisitive educational approach.

I got to know Jack personally while working as editor of the *Feldenkrais* Journal, the professional publication for the *Feldenkrais* community. Jack authored a number of articles and joined the editorial board in the 1980s. One thing I greatly appreciate about Jack was that when he offered an opinion or contribution it was always fresh, always a departure from what everyone else was saying. He was a man who thought for himself and had his own, sometimes idiosyncratic, ideas on a wide range of subjects. Not everyone agreed with him or his approach, but no one could argue with the effectiveness of his work. He could walk the talk.

Jack was also very interested in athletics, seriously pursuing karate, skiing, golf and running at various times. He organized his life for more than a decade so he could spend a large part of the winter skiing, packing all his clients into a few workdays so he could spend most of the week skiing. Jack wrote extensively on applying the *Feldenkrais Method* to sports, authoring Running with the Whole Body and various articles for professional journals. He also put together a number of CD programs that sell widely: Total Body Golf, Running with the Whole Body, Total Body Vision and A Healthy Back in Less Than 20 Minutes.

Jack passed away on May 10, 2002. Jack is remembered fondly by many and his influence continues, especially through his writings and CD programs that are widely appreciated.

Elizabeth Beringer
San Diego, California
June 19, 2011

Introduction

The eyes are probably the most important and yet the least understood of man's sensory organs. Consider the way that we test the eyes by "reading the eye chart." If, from a certain distance we are able to recognize the familiar shapes of the letters on the chart, our eyes are all right. If not, glasses or contacts are prescribed so that we can read.

Of course, an orthodox eye care professional will do a much more extensive test, but mostly he is testing your ability to read. Is this all that there is to vision?

There is good reason to believe that reading—that is, recognizing previously memorized shapes—is only a small part of what the visual system does, and that from the standpoint of good overall use of the body and mind, reading is of lesser importance than the other functions of the visual system. These other functions of the visual system are chiefly concerned with movement. In fact, organizing the body for movement is the chief function of the visual system.

A minute or two of reflection on the evolutionary heritage of our species gives support to this position. For millions of years our animal and human ancestors depended on their eyes to capture prey, or to avoid being captured themselves. To accomplish this, the eyes must be able to sense position and velocity with respect to the body with extreme precision and speed, and to direct movement toward or away from prey or predator, as the case may be, instantly.

There is considerable evidence that reading and this other use of the eyes are organized by different subsystems within the visual system. In rare cases of injury, it is possible for one subsystem to work when the other has been destroyed.

In his book, *Languages of the Brain*, Dr. Karl Pribram, the Stanford neuropsychologist, describes cases of what he calls blind sight, where an individual with central nervous system injury cannot "see" an object (that is, he cannot name it), but can point to it. Therefore, many of the functional connections concerned with movement, between the eyes and the body, are outside of conscious awareness.

If you have ever taken one more or one less step at the top or bottom of a flight of stairs than was actually there, you have experienced a malfunctioning of this part of the visual system. The results can be disconcerting, or even dangerous, if they lead to a fall.

Other clues to the functioning of the visual system, and methods of improving it, are provided by experiments on human subjects with inverting prism glasses, also reported by Dr. Pribram. Subjects who are not allowed to move about and manipulate their environment, never learn to see right side up. So, to improve vision, we must compare visual and kinesthetic information while moving.

One additional item of interest reported by Dr. Pribram concerns the concept that perception consists of an organism forming an internal representation of its environment. Thus, if we can find a way to compare our internal representation of the environment with the environment itself, in such a way that we can cause the internal representation to make a closer match with the environment, we will be improving the internal representation.

In his book *Awareness Through Movement*, Dr. Moshe Feldenkrais makes the point that we act in accordance with our self image. This self image is an internal representation of the body and its relationship to the environment. By improving our internal representation, we can improve the quality of our action.

This use of the eyes in movement is of great importance for individual well-being and good overall use of the body and mind, but it is practically unrecognized in our society. Reading is considered to be so important -indeed, written information is the foundation of our culture -that the use of the eyes in movement is virtually ignored. If vision is not good -that is, if we cannot read the eye chart -we wear glasses to be able to read better, but this severely compromises the use of the eyes in movement.

Working with the eyes in movement can be a very powerful way of improving the functioning of the whole nervous system. There are a number of reasons for this.

First, the area of the brain devoted to processing visual information is unusually large. If we improve the functioning of this large area, the improvements will tend to diffuse throughout the entire brain.

Second, the eye is important as an output device. We usually think of the eye as a sensory organ only, but there are many direct functional connections between the muscles of the eyes and the state of contraction of other muscles in the body. Thus, the eyes are used as both input and output, or sensory and motor devices, in a way that no other sensory organ is used.

Finally, the eye is the initiator of many if not most of our actions. A sequence of actions, such as picking up an object, opening a door, walking across a room, shaking hands, hitting a ball, or starting a parallel turn, begins with fixing something in our visual field. Thus, if the use of the eyes is faulty, all of our movements get off to a bad start. If we can improve this initial action, subsequent movements are then more open to change.

This book consists of a series of exercises to improve the use of the eyes in movement. And because of the fact that all the functions of the nervous system interact with each other, this will improve what we ordinarily call vision -that is, visual acuity also, along with our posture, breathing, movement and thinking.

The basic ideas behind the exercises are drawn from two sources. The first source is the *Awareness Through Movement* system of Moshe Feldenkrais, D.Sc. Each chapter in the book is organized as an *Awareness Through Movement* lesson, and employs the learning principles developed by Dr. Feldenkrais over a period of many years.

The second source, and the original inspiration for trying to improve the use of the eyes, is the work of William H. Bates, M.D. Dr. Bates was the first person to clearly understand that the functioning of the eyes could be improved, and to develop a practical system to do so.

In his book, The Cure of Imperfect Sight by Treatment Without Glasses, published in 1920, Dr. Bates sets forth his ideas on improving vision. One fact, which is not well known, and not mentioned in the book, is that Dr. Bates used some kind of manipulations of the head, neck, spine and pelvis in his treatment of those with defective vision. If any reader of this book knows anything about these manipulations, I would very much like to hear from him or her, through Woodstone Books.

Most of the exercises presented here are my own invention, although some are slight modifications of ones developed by Dr. Bates, or his students. The chapter entitled "Sunning and Palming" is, of course, taken directly from the work of Dr. Bates, although I have added some procedures of my own here, also.

How to do the exercises

Ideally, you should devote two or three sessions of one hour each, per week, to the exercises. After you have read the preliminary material in Chapters One and Two, begin your first session with the exercise in Chapter Three. The next session do the exercise in Chapter Four, the next, Chapter Five, and so on. When you have finished all eleven exercises, return to Chapter Three, and repeat. After a period of time, your vision will improve enough so that you can taper off, doing the exercises less and less frequently, and finally you should arrive at a point where you do not need the exercises at all, or only very infrequently. If your visual system is well organized, your day to day life should provide you with enough exercise for your eyes.

The first time that you do an exercise, be sure to give yourself plenty of time to read and understand the instructions. After that, you will probably find that about an hour to an hour and fifteen minutes will suffice to do one exercise.

Be sure to do the exercises in a well lighted, comfortable room. Have a clear area on the floor, with a rug, so that you can lie down and palm your eyes comfortably, and so that you can have plenty of room to do the exercises that require you to lie on the floor.

No matter what you are doing, be sure to avoid any kind of strain as you do the exercises. Good vision is effortless, and if you are straining, you are just practicing poor vision, and you will not improve. If you find that one of the exercises produces some discomfort, or unusual tiredness, reduce the amount of time spent on each move, or stop completely, and come back to the exercise later. The second or third time around, you will find that you have no trouble.

Finally, when you have finished with an exercise, spend a little while doing something that does not require a concentrated use of the eyes. Go for a walk, or engage in conversation with friends.

Materials

A few supplies, easily obtained at drug stores, office supply stores, etc, are required to do the exercises in this book. They are:

- An eye patch.
- A box of colored push-pins.
- A wooden yard stick. (Get the high quality kind, with brass ends, and check to make sure that it is perfectly straight by sighting along the edge.)
- A *convergence card*. Get a business card, and copy the pattern shown below onto the back of the card. Make the cut out area (cross hatched) just as large as the thickness of the yard stick, so that it will sit on the stick without falling. When you copy the pattern, be certain to make a very exact copy, with the circles positioned in a symmetrical fashion about the mid line, or you will give yourself eye strain when you use the card.

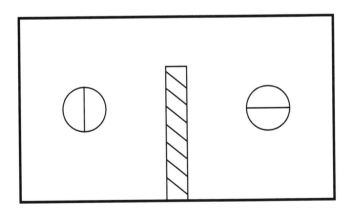

1. Sunning and palming

Sunning and palming are two procedures introduced by Dr. Bates that are indispensable to any program for improving the use of the eyes. Five to ten minutes of sunning, followed by an equal amount of palming, practiced daily, can make quite a difference in the use of the eyes.

Sunning consists of exposing the eyes to direct sunlight in a certain way. This should be done gradually, over a period of weeks, or even months, so as to avoid strain. In particular, if you habitually wear tinted glasses, you should approach sunning in a very slow and gradual way.

To begin, pick a time in the morning or the evening when the sun is not too high above the horizon. Sunning may be practiced at any time that the sun is visible, but it is somewhat awkward to do when the sun is very high in the sky.

Remove glasses or contacts if you wear them, and stand facing the sun. Close your eyes, and begin to turn your whole body left and right, in an easy twisting motion. Your feet remain where they are on the ground.

Continue to turn, and notice the sensations of light and dark in the eyes. As you turn to the right, the left eye will perceive a bright, diffuse, field of light, but the right eye will see a darker field. Then, as you turn to the left, the left eye will see a darker field, and the right eye a brighter one.

As you turn, notice the sensations of warmth on the face and eye lids. Let your attention move slowly through your body, and notice how your feet tilt left and right on the ground, and how your legs and hips turn, and your shoulders and head. Notice your breathing. Is it slow and easy?

When you first begin to do sunning, spend only a few minutes at it, and keep your eyes completely closed. Gradually, begin to spend a longer and longer time, until you have worked your way up to about ten minutes. If at any time you experience any pain or discomfort, cut back on your time.

After a few days or weeks of this, you can begin to open your eyes, one at a time, as follows.

Begin to sun your closed eyes, as described above, and after two or three minutes, open one eye, directed a little below the horizon, and continue to turn left and right. As you turn, slowly raise the eye up so that you look a little above the horizon, then move the eye back down, until you are looking below the horizon. Repeat for one to two minutes.

Then, close that eye, and continue to turn with the eyes closed for another minute. Then, open the other eye and sweep it up and down in the same way as the first eye.

Again close both eyes, and turn left and right for a minute, then open the first eye, sweep it up and down, close it, and sun both closed eyes, and then open the other eye for a minute and sweep it up and down. Finish with a minute of sunning with both eyes closed.

If you experience any discomfort or strain while doing this, close your eyes, and spend a few more days sunning with your eyes closed.

If you continue to have difficulty, stand in the shade and face away from the sun when you first open your eyes. Then, gradually increase the amount of light and the time spent until you can face the sun.

Over a period of weeks, gradually begin to lift your eyes higher and higher, until you can sweep your eye directly across the sun. At this point, you can begin to open both eyes at once, and sweep them left and right just below the horizon. Eventually, you can arrive at a point where it is possible to sweep both eyes directly across the sun, but it is not a good idea to stare directly at the sun.

The idea is sometimes expressed that sunlight is harmful to the eyes, but this like saying that food is harmful to the stomach, or air harmful to the lungs. The eyes require full, natural sunlight to function effectively.

In my personal experimentation with sunning, I spent a winter skiing, and over a period of weeks I worked my way up to a point where I was able to ski for two continuous days in full sunlight, without a single cloud being visible, at an altitude of about ten thousand feet. The sunlight reflected from the white snow makes this one of the most intense natural light environments on earth. At the end of the second day, I experienced some mild discomfort, and a slight reddening of the eyes, and so I finally settled on wearing sunglasses for a few hours in the middle of the day. However, some of my skiing friends do not own a pair of sunglasses, and go all winter with no eye protection, and have excellent vision.

The key thing to remember when sunning, is to proceed gradually, and not to strain the eyes. Over a period of time, many small changes can add up to make one big one.

After sunning, palm your eyes. Lie on your back, and set one or both feet standing if you find that this is comfortable. Close your eyes, and cover one eye with the palm of the corresponding hand.

Set the small finger edge of the hand against the nose, and cup your palm so that the hand does not touch the eye lid. Slide your hand up and down along the nose a little until you find a place where the hand just fits against the face, as if it were made to go there. Then, take the other hand and cover the other eye in the same way. With the eyes closed, and covered by the palms of the hands in this way, no light should be visible. If some light gets in, move your hands around some more until you find the place where the hands block out all light.

After you have covered your eyes, pay attention to any visual sensations. Since the eyes are closed and covered, and no light is coming into them, you would expect to see a uniform field of featureless black. However, many people, especially those with poor vision, see something other than black. This shows that the visual system is indicating an input, when none is there. In the initial exercises, you will cover one eye with an eye patch, and work the other eye for a period of time, and then lie down and palm your eyes. At this point, you can compare the eye that has been worked with the eye that has not, and notice which eye sees a more uniform blackness. Sometime, the effect can be striking.

This is all that there is to palming. You do not have to do anything, just lie still and let your eyes have a rest.

Begin each exercise in the book with a period of sunning and palming, as directed. If you have to do the exercises at a time when the sun is not visible, substitute an incandescent bulb for the sun. Hold your eyes about four to six inches away from the bulb, and turn your head left and right. However, do not open your eyes when you do this. And of course, be sure to get in a few minutes of sunning with the sun itself at some other time during the day.

2: The dominant eye

The large majority of people in our society are either right handed or left handed. That is, they have a dominant hand. Most people also have a dominant eye, which is used preferentially, just like the dominant hand. This eye is used to aim a rifle, or to sight through a telescope.

Here are two ways to determine your dominant eye. One can be done alone, and one requires the help of a friend. Both are worth trying.

To determine your dominant eye by yourself, hold one thumb out at arms length, and sight over it at some object that is at least ten feet away. Make sure that you are looking at the target object. Then, open and close one eye, and then open and close the other eye.

When you open and close the dominant eye, the thumb will appear to jump out of line with the target object. When you open and close the non-dominant eye, the thumb appears to stay in line with the target. (if you pay close attention, you will be able to notice that with both eyes open and focused on the target object, you see two thumbs. Usually the visual system suppresses the image of the thumb from the non-dominant eye, but it is fairly easy to see the "second thumb" if you look for it.)

To determine your dominant eye with the help of a friend, proceed as follows. Have your friend stand about ten feet away, and close one of his eyes. Hold your thumb out at arms length, and sight over your thumb at your friend's open eye. Your friend should look back over your thumb at your face, and he will see your thumb lined up over your dominant eye.

Try both of these ways of determining your dominant eye. Do you come out with the same eye each time?

In the exercises, which begin in the next chapter, we will begin with the dominant eye, and work that eye by itself for a period of time, and then we will work with the non-dominant eye. This arrangement allows the non-dominant eye, which usually has the poorer vision, to learn from the dominant eye.

3: Standing and turning

In our day to day movements, we habitually use our eyes and our legs in particular patterns of motion. Typically, we guide our legs with the dominant eye, and use only a few of the many possible combinations of movement patterns between the eyes and the legs. By exploring some of these unused patterns we can expand the range of movement, and improve our balance, posture, and vision.

To begin the exercise, take off your glasses or contacts, if you wear them, and do about five to ten minutes of sunning. Then, lie on your back and set one or both feet standing flat on the floor with the corresponding knee bent, if you find this comfortable. Close your eyes, and cover them with the palms of the hands, in the way that you have learned.

Take a few minutes and notice what you see -or rather, what you don't see, since there is no light coming into the eyes -with each eye. In particular, compare the left and right visual fields. Do they extend to the sides an equal amount? How about up and down? Are the two visual fields equally black? Move your eyes around a little. Do the eyes feel as if they move easily in the sockets?

Now, stand up facing a blank wall about five or six feet away, and cover the non-dominant eye with an eye patch. Begin to turn the entire body left and right with an easy twisting motion. Your feet remain where they are on the floor. As you turn, imagine that there is something to the left side that you wish to see, then to the right, then left, and so on. Turn your eye to the side and let the body follow, so that the eye leads the motion. Continue to do this and, while paying attention to the visual field, scan your body with your attention. Begin at your feet, noticing how the pressure shifts left and right as you turn, then notice your ankles, calves, knees, thighs, hips, spine, chest, shoulders, head, and eyes. Does the shift of attention change the motion at all? Take three or four minutes to do this.

Continue to turn and close both eyes. Does this change the quality of the turning movement at all? Turn several times with your eyes closed, and then several times with your eyes open, and compare the two movements. With many people, opening the eye actually interferes with the turning movement, instead of guiding it, especially with the non-dominant eye. If you find this to be the case, come back and repeat this initial motion after you have finished the whole exercise, and you will be surprised at the change.

Turn all the way to the right, and stop. Keeping your body still, turn your head and eyes back to the left, and look to the left, then turn the head and eyes to the right again, and look to the right, then left, and so on. Turn the head and eyes left and right like this about ten times, slowly, and then resume the turning motion of the whole body, as you were just doing. Do you turn a little further now? Turn to the left and stop, and again turn the head and eyes right and left about ten times, letting yourself breathe easily. Finally, turn the whole body left and right, letting the eye lead the motion.

Now, shift all of your weight onto your right foot, and continue turning left and right, letting the eye lead the motion. Again scan your body, feet to head, while noticing what you see. After several minutes, shift your weight onto your left foot, and repeat. Notice how the right and left hips move differently when the weight is on one foot.

Continue to turn left and right, and now shift your weight onto your left foot as you turn left, and onto your right foot as you turn right. Then, after a few minutes of this, reverse the weight shift so that your weight goes onto your right foot as you turn left and onto your left foot as you turn right. Remember to notice what you see as you turn, and to let the eye lead the motion. Stop and rest for a minute, without removing the eye patch.

Now, push a colored push-pin into the wall right in front of yourself at eye level, about five or six feet away. Continue to turn left and right as before, but make this change: fix your eye on the push pin so that the eye remains still in space. This requirement of keeping the eye fixed on the target will limit the ability of the head and body to turn.

Notice how the eye stands still and the head turns around it -just the opposite of the way that the head and eye usually move. Continue to turn left and right, and as you turn, begin to pick out objects at the extreme left and right, and top and bottom, of your visual field. The eye remains fixed on the pin as you do this. You should find that, after a few minutes, you can see quite a few objects without making out details. Continue to turn left and right, noticing your entire visual field, and scan your body, feet to head, as before. You may find that it is tricky to pay attention to bodily sensations and visual input simultaneously at first, but if you persist without straining, it will become easy. What else can you see as you turn? How about your nose?

Continue this motion and shift your weight to your right foot as before, for a few minutes, and then to your left foot. Then, shift to the right as you turn right, and to the left as you turn left. Finally, shift your weight right as you turn left and left as you turn right, all the while keeping the eye fixed on the target and scanning the body with your attention.

Notice how this kind of peculiar motion allows you to move the eye muscles and the rest of the body, while at the same time maintaining a constant visual input. This allows you to check and improve the use of the peripheral vision while moving. You will find .that this a very different proposition from a static check, which you can do by having someone wave a light or colored object off to one side while you stand still and look straight ahead.

Now, release the eyes and turn left and right in the easiest way, as in the beginning. Notice how the turning angle of the body has increased. Can you feel just what has changed in your body to enable it to turn further without more effort? Again, stop and rest briefly, without removing the patch.

Resume turning left and right, but now fix both the head and eye on the target. The head and eye remain fixed in space, and the body turns left and right below them. Again, pay attention to the entire visual field, picking out objects at the extreme edge, and slowly scan your body. After a few minutes shift your weight to your right foot, then to your left foot, and then left and right in the two ways that you have learned.

If you pay careful attention to yourself, you may be able to discover an interesting correlation between your awareness of your peripheral visual field, and something that goes on in your mind. What happens when you forget about the peripheral visual field, and then when you remember to pay attention to it again? Can you notice any change in your hearing when you do this?

Release the head and eyes, and let everything turn left and right as before. Notice how the turning angle has increased even more.

Lie on your back, remove the eye patch, close your eyes, and cover them with the palms of your hands as before. Compare the left and right visual fields and notice the difference in what you don't see with the eye that was open, and what you don't see with the eye that was covered. Which eye feels better? Which visual field is blacker? Which field extends further to the sides, and up and down? Move your eyes around under your palms. Which eye moves easier? Notice your breathing. Is there a difference in the breathing movements and the sensation of lung capacity on the left and right sides? Sit up, open your eyes and look around you. What do you see?

Now stand up, cover the dominant eye, and go through the whole exercise again, from the beginning, using the non-dominant eye. Try to time the motions so that the entire sequence takes about 45 minutes to an hour.

When you are finished, stand up and look around. Pay attention not only to what you see, but also to the sensations in the eyes themselves, and to the muscles in the face just around the eyes. Look in the mirror. How does your face look?

If you wear glasses or contacts, put them on and again check the sensation around the eyes. How does it feel now?

From time to time, over the next few days, think about opening your peripheral vision, as you did in the exercise. You can try it in a movie, in a noisy restaurant, while writing, or while walking down the street. Notice the effect. If you are moving, can you detect some change in the quality of your movement when you open your peripheral vision? If you are in a place with a lot of sound, does the quality of your hearing change?

Notes

4: Eyes, neck, and shoulders

In order for the eyes to move easily, the motion of the eyes must be properly coordinated with the motion of the head. The neck muscles, of course, turn the head, but there are also many direct muscular connections between the head and the shoulders. Thus, proper eye movement depends in part on the organization of the whole upper body. In this chapter we are going to work to improve this organization.

As usual, do about five minutes of sunning and then five minutes of palming. Then, sit down on the floor, and turn your head left and right a few times. Notice how far the head turns, and how easily. Get a good feeling for the motion of the head so that you will be able to feel the improvement at the end of the exercise. Then, find a space with a rug, and lie down flat on your back, arms and legs stretched out comfortably on the floor. Notice how your body lies on the floor, and which parts make contact with the floor, and which parts do not.

As you lie there, draw up your knees, so that your feet are standing flat on the floor near your buttocks, and your knees are pointing toward the ceiling. Then, interlace your fingers and put your hands behind your head, palms up, so that the back of the head rests in the cup formed by the hands.

From this position, slowly raise the head a little way off the floor, helping with the arms, and then lower the head back to the floor. Repeat this move several times, and let your elbows rise up and come close together as the head lifts, and then separate and go back to the floor as the head goes down. Repeat this move about ten or fifteen times, moving slowly, and make sure that you do not hold your breath.

Now lift the head up such a small amount that you can still feel the nap of the rug with the back of your hands, and let the elbows rise up and come close together so that the forearms touch the ears. In this position the head is suspended in a cradle formed by the arms and hands.

Very slowly, turn the head a little to the left, and then come back to center. Repeat this move, and let the arms and hands help the head. As the head turns left, the right elbow will go up toward the ceiling a little, and the left elbow will go down toward the floor. Don't let the head slide against the hands. Turn the head left and back to the middle about ten or fifteen times, and then stop, and let the head and elbows rest on the floor.

After resting for about a minute, lift the head and elbows up again, so that the head is suspended in the cradle formed by the hands and arms. This time, turn the head a little to the right, and then come back to center. Repeat this move, turning the head a little to the right and then coming back to center, about fifteen times, and notice how the left elbow goes up and the right elbow goes down as the head turns right.

As you move, pay attention to the quality of the movement, and not just the quantity. Don't turn your head as far as you can, or you will reduce your sensitivity to the point where you cannot feel what you are doing, and you will not get much improvement in the movement of the head and eyes. Again, lower your head and arms to the floor and rest for a minute.

Once again lift the head and elbows up just off the floor, and this time turn the head left and right, without stopping in the middle. As before, let the arms move to help the head. Repeat the motion about ten or fifteen times, and then stretch out your arms and legs and rest on your back.

As you lie there, notice the feeling of the contact of the head and upper body against the floor. Can you feel any change there from the movements that you just made?

After about a minute, draw up your knees, feet standing as before, and interlace your fingers behind your head. Lift the head up a tiny bit, helping with the arms, and turn the head to the left a little. From here, move the eyes left and right, keeping the head still.

As you turn the eyes, let your attention move down to your neck and chest, and notice if you can feel anything there. Do you hold your breath as you move your eyes? Can you feel anything moving in your upper back, around the shoulder blades? Turn the eyes left and right about fifteen times and then stop, lower the head and arms back to the floor, and rest.

Once again lift your head up a little bit, so that it is suspended just off the floor in the cradle of the arms and hands, and turn the head a little to the right. Leaving the head facing to the right, move the eyes to look to the left and right about fifteen times. As before, notice what goes on in the rest of your body as you move your eyes. In particular, make sure that you do not hold your breath. After you are finished, lower the head and arms back to the floor, and rest for a minute.

Now lift the head up a little way as before, and just turn the head left and right, helping with the arms. Notice how the head turns further and with less effort than at the beginning of the exercise. Set the head and arms on the floor, stretch out your arms and legs, and rest for a minute.

Once again, draw up your knees, feet standing comfortably, and interlace your fingers behind your head. Lift your head up a little way, letting the elbows come close together, so that the head is suspended easily in the cradle of the arms.

Now, move the eyes over to the left, so that the pupil of the left eye is at the outside corner of the eye, and the pupil of the right eye is at the inside corner, near the nose. Holding the eyes in this position, turn the head left and right, helping with the arms, as before.

If you have a friend reading to you, have him watch your eyes carefully to be sure that they stay over to the left side.

Many people find that they are unable to do this simple move the first time that they try it. With their eyes turned to the side, they suddenly find that their neck muscles have turned to stone, and they are unable to move their head.

If you experience this, stop and think for a minute about what this means. Imagine that you are running for a tennis ball, or racquet ball, or whatever, and that the ball is off to the side and that you must turn your eyes to the side to see it. With your eyes turned to the side, you immobilize your neck muscles and hold your breath, just as you did while lying on the floor. With a large part of the muscles of your body tied up fighting each other like this, what kind of shot are you going to make?

some people spend years trying to learn a sport, and never become very good at it. Finally, they resign themselves to being a permanent beginner, or even give up and quit altogether, telling themselves "i'm not coordinated," or something like that. Actually, the problem is just a lack of awareness of how the various parts of the body work together, and it can be corrected with just a few hours of easy movement.

Spend a few minutes playing with this move. Hold your eyes over to the left, take a breath, and slowly let it out. As you breathe out, begin to turn the head left and right, helping with the hands and arms. As you move, think about your neck, and your chest and shoulders, and your tongue and jaw. Do you tighten any of these parts of yourself as you turn your head? As you begin to think of these different parts, you will find that the motion of turning the head becomes smooth and easy.

Continue this same turning motion, but close your eyes. Does this make it more or less easy to turn the head? Open your eyes, and turn the head left and right, still keeping the eyes turned to the left. Then turn a few more times with the eyes closed, then open, and so on.

When the eyes are open, we tend to fix the eyes by sighting on some object. When the eyes are closed, we must fix them by paying attention to the sensations of movement in the eye muscles. Thus, in this motion, most people find it easier to fix the eyes in the sockets with the eyes closed. After comparing the two movements, however, each becomes equally easy.

Set your head and arms down on the floor and rest briefly. Then, raise the head up again, helping with the hands, and move the eyes over to the right. Holding the eyes to the right, again turn your head left and right. Be sure to let the elbows move up and down as the head turns. Experiment with the eyes open and closed, as you did when the eyes were turned to the left. After about fifteen turns, lower your head and arms to the floor and rest for a minute.

Once more lift your head up just off the floor, helping with the arms and hands. Begin to turn the head left and right. As the head turns to the left, move your eyes to the right, and, as the head turns to the right, move your eyes to the left. Make another fifteen moves like this, turning the eyes in the direction opposite to the direction of the head.

Lower your head and arms to the floor and rest briefly. Then, lift your head and arms up as before, and just turn the head left and right in the easiest way, without doing anything in particular with the eyes. How does the head motion feel now? Probably a lot easier. Put your head down, stretch out your arms and legs, and rest for a minute.

As you lie there, notice how your head and shoulders, and your whole back, lie against the floor. Is there some change from when you began the exercise?

Draw up your knees and interlace your fingers behind your head as before. Lift your head up a tiny bit, helping with the hands, and let the elbows come up so that they point to the ceiling.

From this position, begin to swing the head and arms left and right so that the head moves from side to side on the floor, but the nose continues to face the ceiling.

Notice that this is a completely different move from what we have been doing up to now. In the first part of the exercise, the head stayed in one place, and turned left and right. Now the head does not turn, but instead moves over to the left side and then back to the right, so that the head swings in an arc on the floor, and the elbows remain at the same level.

Make about fifteen moves like this; swinging the head left and right, and keeping the nose pointing to the ceiling. Then, bring the head to the center, and once again turn the head left and right, so that the eyes face first one side, and then the other, and the elbows move up and down.

Go back and forth between these two moves -swinging the head and turning the head -until you can do each easily. You will find that as you become clear about the difference between the two moves, that each move actually becomes easier to do. Notice that when you turn the head, the eyes face to the left and right, and the elbows move up and down, but the head remains over the same point on the floor. When you swing the head, the eyes face straight up toward the ceiling, and the elbows do not move up and down, but the head moves to the right and left in an arc on the floor. Put your head on the floor, stretch out your arms and legs, and rest.

Once again set your feet standing, and interlace your fingers behind your head. Lift the head up a tiny bit, helping with the hands. From this position, slide the head to the left while turning it to the right, and then reverse the motion, and slide the head right while turning it left. Continue to do this for about fifteen or twenty repetitions, and then bring the head to the center, set it down, and stretch out and rest.

Set your feet standing, interlace your fingers behind your head, and raise your head up a little bit, helping with the hands. Open your eyes, and look at a point on the ceiling directly overhead. Keeping the eyes fixed on the spot, turn the head left and right. Turn the head about fifteen times, and then close the eyes, and continue turning the head. Is the head motion easier with the eyes closed? Continue to turn the head, and open the eyes and again look at the same spot. Does this interfere with the motion of the head?

Keep turning the head left and right like this, making a few moves with the eyes open and fixed on the spot, and then a few moves with the eyes closed and relaxed, then with the eyes open, and so on. After a few repetitions of this sequence, you will find that the head turns as easily with the eyes open and fixed on the spot as it does with the eyes closed. Stop moving, stretch out and rest. Notice how your body lies against the floor. Are different areas in contact with the floor than when you began the exercise? Notice the sensation of breathing in the upper chest. Is the motion larger than usual?

After resting for a minute, roll over to one side, and sit up. Slowly turn your head left and right, as you did at the beginning. Notice how much further the head turns, and how much easier. Stand up and look around. How is the clarity of your vision?

Walk around a little. How does it feel to walk? Breathe into your upper chest. How does that feel? Can you determine how moving your head and eyes in different ways can improve your breathing like this?

5: Eyes left/right

For efficient use of the eyes in movement, the motions of the eyes must be properly coordinated with the motions of the head, neck, spine, and pelvis. In the previous lesson, we began to work with this coordination while lying down, and we concentrated mainly on the sensations of movement in the eyes themselves. In this lesson, we are going to work with this coordination while sitting, and we will work with visual input along with kinesthetic sensations. Also, we will begin to compare our internal visual representation of the world, with the real world outside, and by so doing, we will improve the internal representation. Since this internal representation guides our movements, improvements there will be reflected in improved movement.

Take off your glasses or contacts if you wear them, and then do about five minutes of sunning, and then five minutes of palming. As you palm your eyes, compare the extent of the left and right visual fields, and notice if each side is a uniform, featureless, black.

When you have finished palming, sit in a chair with a flat, horizontal seat. The height of the chair should be such that your feet rest flat on the floor, and your hips and knees are bent at right angles. Arrange the chair so that you face a section of blank wall, from about five or six feet away.

Take your yardstick, and stick a pushpin into the long, narrow side, just at the end of the stick. Cover your non-dominant eye with the eye patch. Hold the yardstick at one end, with the pushpin at the other and about at eye level. Wave the stick left and right, and look at the pin as it moves. Try moving the stick slowly, and then faster, and in a small arc and then a larger one. Can you follow the pin easily, or do you feel as if it takes some effort to do so?

Now, hold the yardstick horizontally, with one end touching your face just below the uncovered eye, and the stick pointing straight out in front. The pin is at the far end of the stick, pointing to the ceiling, and the hand supporting the stick is about eight to twelve inches away from your face. When you first do this exercise, make sure that the wall beyond the stick is blank, so that your eyes are not distracted. Later, you can try the exercise with a visually rich background, such as a bookshelf, beyond the pin, and improve even more.

Sit facing straight toward the wall, and hold the stick straight out in front, touching your face. Have a friend stand behind you and observe the configuration of your body, the wall, and the stick. Does your friend see the stick as being "straight out in front?" (that is, perpendicular to the wall?) With many people, the visual sensation of "straight out in front" is twenty or thirty degrees to one side, and it can be different for each eye. If you find that this is the case for your eyes, just take note of the fact, and continue with the exercise. The next time that you do the exercise, check your sensation of "straight out in front" again, and notice if it has changed for the better, so that your internal sensation matches reality.

As you sit there, move the stick so that the pin moves horizontally inward a few inches, and then return the pin to its starting position. If your right eye is open, you will move the pin to the left, and if your left eye is open, you will move the pin to the right. The near end of the stick remains fixed to your face, and the stick pivots about this end. Continue to move the stick, and follow the motion of the pin with your eye only. This means that the head, shoulders, and torso remain fixed, and only the eye moves to follow the pin.

Continue to move the stick and pin inward and back to the center. As you follow the pin with the eye, keep the eye fixed on the pin, but be aware of the peripheral visual field. Notice how the walls of the room swing left and right as the pin moves right and left. Repeat this move for about two or three minutes, and then come back to the center and stop.

From this position, move the pin out, away from the midline, exactly opposite to the motion that you just made. Move the pin out in a horizontal line a few inches, following the pin with a movement of the eye only, and then move the pin back to the mid line. Repeat this move for about two or three minutes, and then stop.

Now move the pin left and right, in a horizontal line, and follow it with your eye. Move the pin a number of times with the eye open, and then close the eye and follow the motion in your imagination. Move the pin left and right a number of times, and visualize the stick and the pin moving. Then, stop moving, open your eye and look at the pin. Are you actually looking at the pin? That is, does your mental picture of the position of the stick and pin match the actual position of the real stick and pin?

When your eye is open, you see the stick and the pin as they really are. When your eye is closed, and you are visualizing the stick and pin, you are seeing your internal representation of the stick and pin. does the imaginary, internal representation of the position of the stick match the position of the real stick?

Notice that when you move the stick with your eye open, you have to pay attention to the visual input from the eye. However, when you move the stick with your eye closed, you have to pay attention to the sensation of motion in the eyeball itself, which is something that we rarely do, and also to the sensations of movement in the hand and arm which are supporting the stick.

Repeat this sequence of tracking the pin with the eye open for a few moves, and then closing the eye and tracking the pin in your imagination. Then, stop moving, open your eye, and notice if the position of the imaginary stick matches the position of the real stick. After a few trials, you will probably find that the real stick and the imaginary stick become one. Stop moving, set the stick down, and rest for a minute.

Once again, hold the stick as you did before, with one end resting against your cheek just under the eye that is open. The stick is horizontal, and the end with the push pin is straight out in front. From this position, turn the entire head, eye, stick and hand together so that you are turning away from the eye that is open. If your right eye is open, for example, turn your head and eye to the left.

The eye continues to look at the pin, and remains fixed in the head as you turn, so that you are tracking the pin by moving the head only. The head, eye, stick and hand turn to the side as if they were one solid piece. The turning motion is in the neck, and the torso remains still. Continue to turn, moving to the side and back to the center, for two or three minutes. The pin needn't move very far, six inches to a foot is enough.

Continue to move, and pay attention to the distance between the chin and the shoulders. Notice how the chin moves closer to one shoulder as the head turns to the side.

Now bring the pin to the midline, and begin to turn it toward the outside, in the opposite direction to the way that you just moved. Continue to turn the head, eye, stick and hand to the side, and pay attention to the sensations of motion in the body, and make sure that you keep your eye fixed on the pin. Spend two or three minutes at this, and then set the stick down and rest.

Once again raise the stick up and hold it as before, and now move the pin left and right by turning the head, eye, stick and hand as a single unit. Spend two or three minutes at this, and be sure to notice what you can see with your peripheral vision as you turn.

Continue to turn, and now close your eyes, and visualize the stick and pin in front of you. Turn left and right two or three times with your eyes closed, and then stop moving, open your eyes, and compare the position of the imaginary stick and pin with the actual position. Then, close your eyes and make a few more movements left and right, then open them, and so on. Is the effect different from when you were tracking the stick with only the eye moving? After two or three minutes of this, put the stick down and rest.

Once again pick up the stick and go back to the position that we have been using, with the stick held straight out in front. Fix your eye on the pin and begin to turn the stick and pin left and right by twisting the torso. In this motion, the eye, head, shoulders, chest, and stick all move as a single unit. The hips remain still on the chair. Notice how the chin remains centered between the shoulders as the body turns.

Continue to turn left and right like this, by twisting the torso, and follow the pin with your eye. Keep your eye fixed on the pin, and notice all the things that you can see with your peripheral vision.

After two or three minutes of turning, close your eyes, and follow the pin for a turn or two with your imagination. Then, stop moving, open your eyes, and compare the position of the imaginary stick with the position of the real stick. That is, you compare your internal representation of the stick, with the real stick. Do this a number of times, and notice how the position of the imaginary stick comes to match the real stick. Stop moving, put the stick down, and rest.

Pick up the stick and hold it as before. Begin to pull your right knee in toward yourself and push your left knee out away from yourself. Then, reverse this movement and pull the left knee in and push the right knee out. Continue to do this, and notice how your pelvis turns left and right on the chair. Let your upper body follow along so that your torso, shoulders, head, eye, and the stick, all turn left and right. As before, keep your eye on the pin.

After a minute of turning, close your eyes and follow the pin in your imagination. After a few turns, stop and compare the position of the imaginary stick with the position of the real stick. Repeat this a few times, and then stop and rest.

Once again, pick up the stick, and hold it in the position that we have been using. This time, keep the hand that is holding the stick still in space, and turn the head left and right a little, so that the nose moves to each side about one or two inches. Notice that as the head turns to the right, the stick pivots about the hand like a horizontal see-saw, so that the pin moves to the left. Then, as the head turns to the left, the pin moves to the right.

Continue to do this, and follow the pin with your eye. This is a different move from the earlier ones that we did, because the eye' must turn in the opposite direction to the head. As you look at the pin, be sure to be aware of your peripheral vision.

After a few minutes of this, close your eyes, and follow the pin in your imagination. As before, open your eyes after a few turns, and compare the imaginary stick with the real stick. Do this several times, and notice if the imaginary stick is in the same place as the real stick. In order to do this, you have to pay attention to the feeling of the end of the stick against your cheek, to the sensation of your hand in space, and to your internal representation of the stick and pin.

Because the head is turning in the opposite direction to the pin, you may find that it takes you several minutes to attain an accurate representation of the motion of the stick with your eyes closed. Remember to breathe from time to time as you do this. When you are finished, put the stick down, and rest.

Once again, pick up the stick, and just wave it left and right, and follow it in the easiest way with your eye, as you did at the beginning of the exercise. Is it easier to follow the pin now? Suppose that instead of a pin you were trying to follow a tennis ball, or a base ball. Would that be easier?

Take off the eye patch, lie down on the floor and cover your eyes with the palms of your hands. As you lie there, compare what you don't see with your left eye with what you don't see with your right eye. Are the two visual fields equally black? Do they extend to the sides an equal amount? How about up and down? Move your eyes around a little, and compare the sensation of movement in the two eyes. Which moves easier? Notice your breathing. Does the breathing motion feel different in the two sides of the chest?

After a few minutes of palming, sit up, open your eyes, and look around. Compare the vision in the two eyes. You will probably notice a peculiar sensation in the vision of the eye that was open, almost as if more light were coming into it, or if the visual field had expanded somehow. What you are sensing is an improvement in your internal representation of the world.

Take your eye patch and cover the other, or dominant eye. Go back through the entire series of motions again, with the non-dominant eye open.

Begin by following the motion of the pin with a movement of the eye only. Follow the pin with the eye open, and then with it closed, as you did earlier.

Then, after a short rest, follow the pin with a motion of the head only, by twisting the neck. Next, follow the pin with a movement of the whole upper body, by twisting the lower torso. Then, follow the pin by moving the pelvis and legs. Finally, keep the hand that is holding the stick still in space, and turn the head left and right, so that the pin moves in the opposite direction to the head. In each case, remember to notice what you see with your peripheral vision, and to do the motion with your eye open, and then closed.

After you are finished, take off the patch and lie down and cover your eyes with the palms of your hands. Compare the left and right visual fields, and the sensations of motion in the two eyes, as you did before. After a few minutes stand up and look around. Do the two eyes seem more equal now?

6: Eyes, neck, and pelvis

In the previous two chapters, we worked with the movement of the eyes to the left and right. In this chapter and the next one, we will work with the movement of the eyes up and down. As before, we will begin by working on the floor, and then finish with sitting.

Take off your glasses or contacts if you wear them, and then do about five minutes of sunning, and then five minutes of palming.

Lie down on your back, with your arms and legs stretched out, and notice how your body makes contact with the floor. Pay particular attention to the head, spine, and pelvis.

Now, draw up your knees so that your feet are standing flat on the floor, comfortably apart. Your arms are lying at your sides.

Push your stomach out a little, arching the small of the back, and notice how the pelvis rolls on the floor so that the point of contact of the pelvis and the floor moves toward the tailbone. Relax and let the pelvis come back to its rest position. Repeat this motion, moving slowly and without straining, and let yourself breathe easily. As you move, notice your head. Does the head move on the floor? If you don't hold your breath, you will find that the head rolls a little on the floor so that the chin approaches the chest as the stomach is pushed out. Continue to roll the pelvis and head like this for two or three minutes. Stop and rest briefly, leaving the feet standing.

Now roll the pelvis the other way, so that the point of contact of the pelvis and the floor moves toward the spine, pushing the small of the back down flat onto the floor. Then, relax and let the pelvis come back to its resting position.

Repeat this motion, moving slowly and without straining, and let yourself breathe easily. Again, notice your head. This time, the head will roll on the floor so that the chin moves away from the chest, as the small of the back flattens out on the floor. Continue to roll the pelvis and head like this for two or three minutes. Stop and rest briefly, leaving the feet standing.

Now, combine the previous two movements, and roll the pelvis up and down on the floor. Let yourself breathe easily, and notice how the head rolls on the floor in a similar manner to the pelvis. When the point of contact of the pelvis and floor moves down toward the feet, the point of contact of the head and floor also moves down toward the feet. Continue to roll up and down like this, and let your attention move slowly along your spine. Notice how the spine moves against the floor. Can you feel all parts of the spine easily, or are there parts of the spine where the sensation of contact of the spine and floor is unclear?

Now, continue to rock the pelvis as before, but stiffen the neck muscles, so that the head slides on the floor. That is, the same point on the head continues to make contact with the floor. Try this for about a minute, and then release the neck muscles, and again let the head roll on the floor. Let the head roll for a minute, then again stiffen the neck muscles and let the head slide, and finally let the head roll easily. Does the movement of the head, spine, and pelvis seem easier now? Stretch out your legs and rest for a minute.

Once again draw up your knees, with the feet standing comfortably flat on the floor. Roll the pelvis up and down on the floor a few times, as you just did, and let the head follow the motion of the pelvis. Now roll the pelvis up so that the small of the back is pressed against the floor, and the chin is away from the chest. Stop in this position.

Holding this position, move the eyes up and down so that you look up toward your forehead, and then down toward your feet. Continue to do this, and make sure that your eyes trace out a straight line as they move up and down. Move the eyes like this for about twenty repetitions, letting yourself breathe easily. Can you feel your back muscles moving as you move your eyes? Stop and rest, leaving the feet standing.

Begin to roll the pelvis up and down, and after a few rolls stop with the small of the back lifted up, and the chin close to the chest.

Holding this position, move the eyes up and down as if to look at the forehead and then at the feet, about twenty times. Again, make sure that the eyes trace out a straight line as they move. Pay attention to the muscles of your back as you move your eyes. Can you feel anything here as you move your eyes? Release your eyes, and just roll the pelvis and head up and down in the simplest way. Is the motion easier now? Stop moving, stretch out, and rest.

Once again draw up your knees, so that your feet are standing. Roll your pelvis and head up and down about ten times. Now, continue to roll, but move your eyes as if to look up at your forehead, and hold them there. What does this do to the rolling motion of the head and pelvis? Hold your eyes up like this and make about ten up and down movements of the pelvis and head, and then release the eyes, and continue to roll the pelvis and head.

Many people find that holding the eyes in this position actually interferes with the free movement of the head, neck, and spine. That is, the eyes and the body do not work with each other, but against each other. Sometimes, the neck muscles become completely immobilized, and the head stops rolling, and begins to slide on the floor.

Continue to move, and make about ten up and down movements of the pelvis and head with the eyes looking up toward the forehead, and then release the eyes and do another ten up and down movements. Repeat this sequence several times, letting yourself breathe easily, and paying attention to the sensations of movement in the back, and you will find that the up and down rolling movement of the head and pelvis will become equally easy with the eyes looking up, or with the eyes relaxed. Stop and rest for a minute, leaving your feet standing.

Now move your eyes and look down. Holding your eyes in this position, roll the pelvis and head up and down as before. Do the eyes interfere with the movement in this position? As before, make about ten up and down movements of the pelvis and head with the eyes looking down, and then another ten with the eyes relaxed, then ten more with the eyes looking, down, and so on.

Finally, just roll the pelvis and head up and down in the easiest way, without doing anything in particular with the eyes. Let the pelvis make the movement, and let the head follow the pelvis passively. Compare the quality and range of the movement now with when you began the exercise. There should be a considerable improvement. Stop moving, stretch out, and rest.

Draw up your knees, feet standing comfortably apart on the floor. Begin to roll your pelvis up and down, and let your head follow the movement. After about ten repetitions, begin to move your eyes in the opposite direction to your head. As your head tilts down, and your chin moves closer to your chest, move your eyes to look up toward your forehead; then, as your head tilts up, and your chin moves away from your chest, move your eyes and look down toward your feet.

Does this movement of the eyes interfere with the free movement of the head and pelvis? It probably will at first. Make about ten up and down movements of the head and pelvis with the eyes moving in the opposite direction to the head, and then release the eyes, and make another ten up and down movements, then again move the eyes in the opposite direction to the head, and so on. After a few rounds of this, you will find that you can move the eyes without interfering with the movement of the head, spine, and pelvis. Stop moving, stretch out your legs, and rest. As you lie there, notice how your body makes contact with the floor. Which parts have changed since you began the exercise? How does your breathing feel?

Draw up your knees, feet standing. Begin to roll the pelvis up and down, as you have been doing, and let the head follow the movement of the pelvis. After a minute, begin to look around at different points on the ceiling. Fix your eyes on some point, and hold them there for a few seconds, then look at another point, and then another, and so on. Does this looking around interfere with the motion of the head and pelvis?

Let the eyes be relaxed, and rock the pelvis up and down a few times, and then look at a few points on the ceiling, then again relax the eyes, and so on. After a few trials you will find that you can use your eyes to look around without interfering with· the movement of the head, spine and pelvis.

We spend much of our waking life looking at this, that, and the other thing, and for many people, the simple act of fixing the eyes on something involves stiffening the muscles of the head, neck, spine, and pelvis, as you probably just felt as you were looking around at the ceiling in the previous movement. Because of this, our spines are much stiffer than they should be. Stop moving, stretch out, and rest. Check your breathing, and the contact of your back with the floor.

After a minute, stand up, and look around. Move your head, eyes, neck, spine and pelvis around some. How do they feel?

7: Eyes up/down

In the previous chapter, we worked with moving the eyes up and down in combination with the head, spine, and pelvis. In this chapter, we are going to do the same thing, except that we will be sitting, and we will pay more attention to visual input.

Take off your glasses or contacts if you wear them, and do about five minutes of sunning, and then lie on your back and do five minutes of palming. As you palm your eyes, move them around a little, left and right, and up and down, and notice the sensation of movement of the eyes. Does the movement feel easy and smooth, or hard and jerky?

When you have finished palming, sit in a chair with a flat, horizontal seat. The height of the chair should be such that your feet rest flat on the floor, and your hips and knees are bent at a right angle. Arrange the chair so that you face a section of blank wall. Make sure that the chair exactly faces the wall, so that the front edge of the chair is parallel to the wall. Sit in the chair so that your hips, shoulders, and head face straight ahead toward the wall.

Cover your non-dominant eye with the eye patch. Arrange the yardstick as in chapter five, with the pushpin stuck into the stick at one end of the long, narrow, side. Hold the yardstick at the other end and wave the pin up and down a few times, and follow the motion of the stick with your eye. Is it easy to follow the motion of the stick?

Now hold the stick up horizontally straight out in front of your face, with the pin away from you. Bring the end that is close to your face in, and hold it against the temple of the eye that is. Open. The wide flat part of the stick should be horizontal, and the pin should be on the part of the stick that faces in toward the midline of the body. With your open eye, you can sight along the narrow edge of the stick and see the pin. With the hand that is on the side of the eye that is open, you will be grasping the stick at a point about eight to ten inches away from your face. Make sure that the stick is straight out in front of your face, so that it is perpendicular to the wall, and not turned off to the right or left at all.

From this point, move the pin down a few inches, by pivoting the stick about your temple, and then move it back up to the starting point. Repeat this motion, and follow the pin with a motion of your eye only. That is, the head and torso remain still, and only the eye moves to track the pin. As you move, pay attention to what else you can see with your peripheral vision. After about two or three minutes, set the stick down and rest briefly.

Bring the stick back to the starting position, and this time move the pin up, by pivoting the stick about the temple, and then move it back down to the starting position. Repeat the motion, and follow the movement of the pin with the eye only. After two or three minutes, stop and rest.

Bring the stick back to the starting position, and now combine the two previous motions, and move the pin up and down. Follow the motion of the pin with a movement of the eye only, and be sure to notice what you see with your peripheral vision. After about a minute or two, close your eye and follow the motion of the pin in your imagination.

Make two or three swings like this, then stop moving, open your eye and notice if you are really looking at the pin. Make a few more up and down moves with the eye open, and then close the eye and track the motion in your imagination, then stop, open the eye, and so on. After several rounds like this, you will find that the position of the imaginary stick that you see with your eyes closed coincides with the real stick. That is, your internal representation of the stick will begin to match the real stick. Set the stick down and rest for a minute.

Once again bring the stick back to the starting position, held horizontally straight out in front. Check to make sure that your hips, shoulders, head and the stick are all facing straight ahead.

Once again tilt the stick in such a way as to move the pin down, and this time follow the pin with a movement of the head only. That is, the eye remains fixed in the head, and the head tilts so as to allow the eye to follow the pin. The head, eye, and stick move as if they were one piece. Repeat this motion for two or three minutes, and think of your breathing from time to time. Stop and rest.

Bring the stick back to the starting position, and this time move the pin up, and follow the motion of the pin with a movement of the head only. Repeat this motion for two or three minutes, and again stop and rest.

Once again bring the stick back to the starting position, and now combine the two previous movements, moving the pin up and down, and follow the movement of the pin with a motion of the head only. Be sure to notice what you can see with your peripheral vision, and make sure that only the head moves, and that the torso is still.

After a few minutes, close the eyes, and follow the motion of the pin in your imagination. Move the pin and stick up and down several times, then stop, open your eyes, and notice if you are really looking at the pin. Repeat this sequence several times, until you find that you are really looking at the pin when you open your eyes. Stop and rest for a minute.

Once again go back to the starting position. Now move the pin down by leaning forward at the hips. The eye, head, neck, and spine all move as a unit, and the eye remains fixed on the pin. Move the pin down by tilting forward at the hips, and then bring the spine back to vertical. Repeat this move for two or three minutes, and then stop and rest.

Bring the stick back to the starting position, and this time move the pin up by tilting the body backward at the hips. As before, the eye, head, spine and stick all move as a unit. Repeat for two or three minutes, paying attention to your breathing, and to what you can see with your peripheral vision. Stop, set the stick down, and rest.

Once again bring the stick back to the starting position, and now combine the two previous motions, moving the pin up and down, by tilting the whole body forward and back so that you pivot about the hip joints. You need not make a large movement with the pin, eight to twelve inches up and down is plenty. As you move, pay attention to the sensation of motion in the body. Can you feel your pelvis rolling forward and back on the chair seat?

After a minute of tracking the pin like this, continue to move, and close your eye, and follow the motion of the pin in your imagination. After several up and down movements, stop, open your eye, and look at the pin. Is the imaginary stick in the same position as the real stick? Repeat this sequence several times, tracking the pin with the eye open, then closing the eye and tracking the pin in your imagination, and then stopping and opening the eye and noticing if you are looking at the pin. After several repetitions of this, you will find that you are really looking at the pin when you open your eye. Stop and rest.

Once again bring the stick back to the starting position. Now move the head forward a little, but keep the head and the stick horizontal. Keep your eye on the pin, and move the head forward and backward with a motion of the neck only. The torso remains still. Continue to do this, and direct your attention to your neck. Can you feel how the neck moves so as to allow the head to move forward and back while remaining horizontal?

As before, do a few motions with the eyes open, and then a few with the eyes closed, and stop and check to see if you· are really looking at the stick. Remember to think of your breathing and to notice what you can see with your peripheral vision. Stop and rest.

Once again go back to the starting position. Move the stick forward a little, until the comer of the stick rests in the notch of bone just at the outside comer of the eye that is open. Nod the head up and down, and notice that as the head tilts down, the pin moves up. Then, as the head tilts up, the pin moves down. The motion of the stick is just like a seesaw, with the hand that is holding the stick acting as the pivot point.

Continue to tilt the head up and down, and follow the motion of the pin with your eye. Let yourself breathe easily, and notice what you can see with your peripheral vision. After a few minutes of this, continue to track the pin with your eyes closed. Go up and down a few times, then stop, open your eyes, and check to see if you are really looking at the pin. Repeat this sequence several times. When your eye is closed, imagine the movement of the whole stick, and your head, and feel just how far the hand that is holding the stick is away from your eye. After several minutes of imaging, stop and rest.

Take off the eye patch, lie on your back, and cover your eyes with the palms of your hands. As you lie there, compare the sensation of blackness in the eye that was open with the eye that was covered. Move the eyes up and down a few times. Which eye moves easier? Notice the breathing movements on the left and right sides of the body. Which side breathes easier?

After about five minutes of palming, roll to one side and sit up. Open your eyes and look around. Compare the quality of vision in the eye that was open with the eye that was closed, by alternately covering first one eye, and then the other. Which eye sees more clearly? Put the eye patch back on your non-dominant eye, and wave the pin and stick up and down a few times, following the movement of the pin with your eye in the easiest way. Is it easier to follow the pin now than it was at the beginning of the exercise?

Now go back and sit in the chair, and cover your dominant eye with the eye patch. Go through the entire exercise again following the motion of the pin with the non-dominant eye.

When you are finished, go outside and walk around a little, and notice what you see. Look at objects in the distance, then at something close to yourself, look left and right, up and down, and so on. How does your vision feel now? Is your posture any different? How about your breathing?

8: Convergence and the rest point

Because our eyes are separate from each other, each eye sees a slightly different view of the world. Ideally, the brain takes these two images and puts them together-or fuses them -to form one image.

This feature of the visual system is the basis for depth perception. To look at an object close by, the eyes must turn in so that each is directed toward the object. To look at an object further away, the eyes turn more out to the side. When both eyes are directed toward a single point, we say that the eyes converge on the point. The visual system is able to get information about how far away an object is from the eyes by measuring the angle that the eyes turn in.

Therefore, the eyes must converge on a single point in order for the brain to be able to fuse the two images properly. If this does not happen, one of the images is suppressed and depth perception is faulty. In today's lesson, we are going to work with convergence and fusion.

Take off your glasses or contacts, if you wear them, and begin with about five minutes of sunning, and then another five minutes of palming. As you palm, compare the left and right visual fields, and move the eyes around a little and notice if the eyes move easily or not.

Find a straight back chair without arms, and with a flat seat, and place the chair so that it faces away from a blank section of wall. The chair should be about six or seven feet away from the wall. Sit backwards on the chair, so that you straddle the back and face the wall. Place the patch on your non-dominant eye, and arrange your body in a comfortable position.

Lean forward slightly, and rest your elbows on the back of the chair. Do this in such a way that you do not have to round your back. Use a pillow or some padding on the chair back if you need it to be comfortable. Mark this position as a kind of reference position that you can go back to during the exercise. Keeping your body still, close your eyes and breathe easily in and out once or twice. Then, open your eyes, and note where the dominant eye is looking. Mentally mark the exact spot on the wall where your eye appears to be looking.

Repeat this procedure several times, closing and then opening your eye, until you know exactly where the eye is looking when it is at rest. This is the rest point of the dominant eye.

Although you would expect the rest point to be more or less straight out in front, and approximately on the same level with the eye, do not be surprised if you find that this is not the case. Sometime the subjective sensation of the center of the visual field, which I call the rest point, is far off to the side. In the most extreme case that i am aware of, a woman with a severe correction reported that her left eye felt as if it were looking about 50 degrees to the left, while an observer could see that the eye was centered in the socket, and appeared to looking straight ahead.

Be sure to keep your body still in the reference position as you find the rest point. If you move your head to one side, the rest point will appear to move to the side an equal amount, and you will not get a clear measurement of the location of the point.

Take your yardstick, and remove any pushpins that you may have in it. Set yourself in your reference position, and let your eye go to its rest point. Sight along the narrow edge· of the stick as if it were a rifle, and you were aiming it at the rest point. The near end of the stick should be about three to six inches away from your eye. Tilt the stick a tiny bit so that you can see the long edge of the stick.

From this position, look at the rest point, and then look at the far end of the stick, and then at the near end of the stick, and then the far end, and then the rest point, and so on. Go back and forth like this, and let your eye glide smoothly up and down the edge of the stick.

If you have the stick lined up properly the eye will not move in its socket as you look at the far end of the stick, and then at the near end. The eye remains still, and only the focus changes from near to far and back. The edge of the stick will actually appear as a point to your eye. An observer watching you would not be able to see the eye move as you look up and down the stick.

Repeat this for about one or two minutes, and notice if your eye looks easily and continuously up and down the stick, or if there are areas that the eye jumps over, or where you do not see the stick clearly. Think of your breathing from time to time. Are you breathing as you look up and down the stick? Stop and rest.

Go back to your reference position, and let your eye go to its rest point on the wall. Take your stick and sight along the stick at the rest point as you just did.

Hold the far end of the stick where it is, and swing the near end of the stick horizontally toward the midline of the body about one or two inches. If your right eye is open, you will move the end of the stick to the left.

Hold the stick still in this position, and look at the rest point, then at the far end of the stick, and then let your eye glide slowly in along the stick until it is looking at the near end. Then, reverse this sequence of moves, letting the eye move out along the stick to the far end, and then look at the rest point on the wall.

Continue this sequence of moves, and notice if the eye glides smoothly along the edge of the stick, or if there are spots that the eye tends to skip over, or places where the eye does not seem to see the stick. Pay attention to what you see, and also notice the muscular sensations of motion in the eye itself. Keep your breathing in the background of your awareness as you do this. Do you hold your breath at the spots where you have difficulty moving your eye along the stick?

In this move, the eye must change focus as it moves from the far end of the stick to the near end, but now it also must turn in a little as it looks at the near end. An observer watching you would see the pupil of the eye move in toward your nose a little and then out again as you sweep your eye from the far end of the stick to the near end, and then back to the far end. Repeat this move for two or three minutes and then rest.

Go back to the reference position, and let your eye go to its rest point. Take the stick and sight along it to the rest point as you did earlier. Hold the far end of the stick where it is, and move the near end of the stick horizontally away from the midline of the body about one or two inches. If your right eye is open, you will move the near end of the stick to the right.

Hold the stick in this position, and look at the rest point, then at the far end of the stick, and then let your eye glide slowly in along the stick until it is looking at the near end. Then, reverse this sequence of moves, let the eye move out along the stick to the far end, and then look at the rest point on the wall.

Continue this sequence of moves, and notice if the eye glides smoothly along the edge of the stick, or if there are spots that the eye tends to skip over, or places where the eye does not seem to see the stick. Notice your breathing as you do this, and also pay attention to the muscles of your face, lips, jaw, tongue, and neck. Do you tense these muscles as you move your eye in and out along the stick? Can you feel the eyeball itself moving as you look up and down the stick?

Now, the eye turns out a little to look at the stick as it moves from the far end to the near end, and an observer watching you would see the eye turn out a little away from your nose as you let the eye move along the edge of the stick. Repeat this move for two or three minutes and then rest.

Go back to your reference position, and let your eye go to its rest point. Take your stick and sight along it at the rest point as you did earlier.

Holding the far end of the stick where it is, move the near end of the stick straight down about one or two inches.

Hold the stick still in this position, and look at the rest point, then at the far end of the stick, and then let your eye glide slowly in along the stick until it is looking at the near end. Then reverse this sequence of moves, letting the eye move out along the stick to the far end, and then look at the rest point on the wall.

Continue this sequence of moves, and notice if the eye glides smoothly along the edge of the stick, or if there are spots that the eye tends to skip over, or places where the eye does not seem to see the stick. As before, pay attention to your breathing, and to the muscles of the face, scalp, and neck, and to the sensations of movement in the eyeball, and avoid any unnecessary tension there.

Repeat this move for two or three minutes, and notice how the eye must turn down a little as it glides from the far end of the stick to the near end. Stop and rest for a minute.

Go back to your reference position, and let your eye go to its rest point. Take your stick and this time sight along the bottom of the stick at the rest point.

Hold the far end of the stick where it is, and lift the near end of the stick straight up about one or two inches.

Hold the stick in this position, and look at the rest point, then at the far end of the stick, and then let your eye glide slowly in along the bottom of the stick until it is looking at the near end. Then, reverse this sequence of moves, letting the eye move out along the stick to the far end, and then look at the rest point on the wall.

As before, repeat this sequence of moves for two or three minutes, and notice if the eye moves smoothly along the stick, and let yourself breathe easily. This time, the eye will move to look up a little as it moves in to look at the near end of the stick. Stop and rest.

Go back to your reference position and close your eyes. Take a breath, open your eye, and check the rest point as you did at the beginning of the exercise. Is the rest point in the same place? Is the sensation of where the rest point is located more precise now? Take off the eye patch, lie on your back, and palm your eyes for about five minutes. As usual, compare the visual sensations and the ease of motion of the two eyes.

Place the patch on your dominant eye, and go back to your chair. Sit in your reference position, and open and close the non-dominant eye several times, and locate the rest point for this eye. Is it fairly close to the rest point of the other eye?

If the two rest points are in different places, it means that you must make some muscular effort to bring the two eyes to converge on a single point before you can fuse the two images. If the rest points are very far apart, it may be that you are unable to bring them together at all. In this case, the visual system suppresses one of the images, and you have no true depth perception.

Go back through the five movement sequences that you just did with the dominant eye, but this time work with the non-dominant eye. Remember that at first you sighted directly along the stick and then looked from the rest point to the near end of the stick and back. Then, you held the near end of the stick a little to the inside while looking far and close. Next, you held the near end a little to the outside. Then, you held the near end of the stick a little lower, and then a little higher. Finally, you checked the rest point and noticed if it was in the same place as when you began the exercise, or if the sensation of exactly where the rest point is located had become clearer.

After you have finished working with the non-dominant eye, take off the patch, lie down on your back, and palm your eyes for about five minutes.

Sit on the chair facing the wall, as before, and get into the reference position that you have been using. Keeping your head and body still, cover your non-dominant eye with one hand. Then, open and close the dominant eye several times, and mentally mark the rest paint on the wall.

Keep your head perfectly still, remove your hand from your non-dominant eye, and cover the dominant eye with one hand. Open and close your non-dominant eye a few times, and mentally mark this rest paint on the wall.

Go back and forth several times, covering first one eye and then the other, until you can see each rest point clearly. Then, set your hands down, and close both eyes. Imagine that each eye is looking at its rest point. Breathe in, and as you slowly let your breath out, open your eyes and let the two rest points come together.

Try this several times, and do not make any effort to force the two rest points to come together. Rather, let yourself breathe easily, and as you open your eyes, pay attention to the muscular sensations from the eyeballs, and from the neck, face, and spine, and avoid any tensions there. After a few tries, you will probably feel the rest points come together without any effort on your part. Sometimes a very tiny wiggling motion of the spine will assist the points to come together.

After trying this several times, stand up and look around. Go outside. How does the world look to you? Is there a sensation of more depth? Is your posture different?

9: Squeezing the eyes

The state of contraction of the muscles around the eyes directly influences the state of contraction of many of the other muscles in the body, particularly the muscles in the neck and spine. In this lesson we are going to work with this connection between the eyes and the rest of the body.

As usual, begin with about five minutes of sunning, and then another five minutes of palming. Then, rest your arms on the floor beside your body, and draw up your knees, so that your feet are standing on the floor comfortably near your buttocks, about shoulder width apart. Have your eyes closed.

Now, squeeze your eyes shut as tightly as you can for a second or two, and then relax your eyes. Continue to do this, and notice if you do anything with your jaw, or your lips, or your tongue as you squeeze your eyes. Notice your breathing. Do you hold your breath as you squeeze your eyes?

Continue to squeeze your eyes, but now do the squeezing in two stages. Squeeze your eyes about half as much as you squeezed them before, pause for a second, and then squeeze them as tightly as you can. Again pause for a second, and then release the squeezing the same way, in two stages. Repeat this motion for about a minute, and then stop, stretch out and rest.

Now, draw up your knees so that your feet are standing comfortably, and interlace your fingers behind your head. Raise the head, helping with the hands, as if you wanted to look down in the direction of your feet. Then lower your head back down to the floor. Repeat this move, slowly, for about a minute, letting yourself breathe out easily as you lift the head. At the end of each move, be sure to set the head and elbows down onto the floor, and cease all effort. Then, start the next move. Stop moving, and set your head and elbows down on the floor.

Now, squeeze your eyes tightly shut, and repeat the previous motion. Notice if squeezing the eyes shut like this affects the lifting of the head in any way. Just squeeze the eyes shut, and raise and lower the head a few times. Does the head lift as far as before? As easily? Do you hold your breath as you lift the head? Set the head down, relax the eyes, and stop moving for a minute.

Once again lift the head, helping with the hands, but do not make any special effort with the eyes. How does it feel to lift the head now? Repeat this motion a few times, and then try it again with the eyes squeezed tightly shut. Set the head down, stretch out, and rest.

Turn and lie on your right side. Stretch your right arm out on the floor overhead, and rest your head on the arm. Have your knees and hips bent at right angles. Place the palm of your left hand on top of your head, so that the tips of the left fingers come close to the right ear. Your left elbow will be pointing straight up toward the ceiling.

From this position, lift the head straight up, helping with the left hand. Lift the head only as far as is easy, and then lower the head and let it rest on the right arm.

Repeat this motion, slowly, and notice how your spine bends in back, and how the ribs on the left side are drawn together, and how the left hip moves up toward the head a little as the head lifts up. After about a minute or two, lower the head down to the right arm, and stop moving.

Now, repeat this motion, but with the eyes squeezed tightly shut. Hold the eyes squeezed, and raise and lower the head, helping with the left hand. Repeat the motion a number of times, and notice if the squeezing of the eyes affects the lifting of the head. Does the head lift as far as before? As easily? Do you hold your breath?

Continue lifting, but with the eyes relaxed. How does it feel to lift the head now? Once more squeeze the eyes and lift the head for a minute. Set the head down, turn and lie on your back, and rest. Notice how your body lies on the floor. Do the left and right sides feel different? Is there a difference in the breathing motions on the two sides?

Turn and lie on your left side. Stretch your left arm out on the floor overhead, and rest your head on the arm. Have your knees and hips bent at right angles. Place the palm of your right hand on top of your head, so that the tips of the right fingers come close to the left ear. Your right elbow will be pointing straight up toward the ceiling.

From this position, lift the head straight up, helping with the right arm. Lift the head only as far as is easy, and then lower the head and let it rest on the left arm.

Repeat this motion, slowly, and notice how your spine bends in back, and how the ribs on the right side are drawn together, and how the right hip moves up toward the head a little as the head lifts up. After about a minute or two, lower the head down to the left arm, and stop moving.

Now, repeat this motion, but with the eyes squeezed tightly shut. Hold the eyes squeezed, and raise and lower the head, helping with the right hand. Repeat the motion a number of times, and notice if the squeezing of the eyes affects the lifting of the head. Does the head lift as far as before? As easily? Do you hold your breath?

Continue lifting, but with the eyes relaxed. How does it feel to lift the head now? Once more squeeze the eyes and raise and lower the head for a minute. Set the head down, turn and lie on your back, and rest. Again, notice how your body lies on the floor, and compare the breathing movement on the left and right sides of the chest.

Turn over and lie on your stomach. Turn your head to face left. Rest your right ear on the back of your right hand, and rest the right hand on the back of the left hand. The palm of the left hand is on the floor.

Slowly, lift the head and right arm a little bit off the floor, then lower them back to the floor. Repeat this movement, using the right arm to help lift the head. As you move, pay attention to your back muscles, and your breathing. Notice your legs. Do the legs tend to lift a little as you raise the head? After a minute or two, set the head down and stop moving.

Now, squeeze your eyes, and repeat the previous motion, holding the eyes squeezed tightly shut as you move. Notice how squeezing the eyes affects the lifting of the head. Does the head lift as far as before? Does the head feel heavier? Do you hold your breath?

After one or two minutes of this, continue to lift the head, but relax the eyes. How does the motion feel now? Once again, squeeze the eyes and lift the head. After a minute, set your head down and rest.

Still lying on your stomach, turn the head to face right, and change the hands over, so that the left ear rests on the back of the left hand, and the left hand rests on the back of the right hand, which is on the floor.

Slowly, lift the head and left arm a little bit off the floor, then lower them back to the floor. Repeat this movement, using the left arm to help lift the head. As you move, pay attention to your back muscles, and your breathing. Notice your legs. Do the legs tend to lift a little as you raise the head? After a minute or two, set the head down and stop moving.

Now, squeeze your eyes, and repeat the previous motion, holding the eyes squeezed tightly shut as you move. Notice how squeezing the eyes affects the lifting of the head. Does the head lift as far as before? Does the head feel heavier? Do you hold your breath?

After one or two minutes of this, continue to lift the head, but relax the eyes. How does the motion feel now? Once again, squeeze the eyes and lift the head. After a minute, set your head down and rest.

Turn your head to the middle, and rest your forehead on the back of your right hand. The palm of the right hand rests on the back of the left hand.

From this position, lift the head and both arms straight up a little, and then lower them back to the floor. Repeat this move for a minute or two, and let the head, hands and arms come up off the floor as if they were one piece. The forehead continues to touch the right hand. Notice your breathing, and how your back moves. Do your feet and knees lift off the floor? They almost certainly will. Let the head and arms come down to the floor, and stop moving for a minute.

Now, repeat the previous motion, but with the eyes squeezed tightly shut. As before, notice how squeezing the eyes affects the lifting motion, and the breathing. After a minute, continue the lifting motion, but with the eyes relaxed. Then, squeeze the eyes again and raise and lower the head. Stop moving, lie on your back and rest.

Draw up your knees and set your feet standing comfortably. From this position, take a fairly deep breath, and then let it out. Repeat the breathing motion several times, and notice how your chest and abdomen move to push the air in and out of your lungs. Continue to breathe like this, but now hold your eyes squeezed tightly shut.

Notice how the squeezing of the eyes affects the movements of breathing. Do you feel the constriction mainly in your chest, or in your abdomen? Breathe in and out five or six times with the eyes squeezed, and then relax the eyes and continue breathing. After another five or six breaths, squeeze the eyes again and continue to breathe. Finally, stretch out your legs and rest. As you lie there, notice your breathing. Does the motion feel different in any way?

Draw up your knees, so that your feet are standing on the floor comfortably near your buttocks. Interlace your fingers behind your head. Slowly, lift your head a little way off the floor, helping with the hands and arms. Let the elbows come closer together as they lift off the floor. Then, reverse the movement, and let the head and arms come back down onto the floor. Repeat this motion several times, and let yourself breathe out easily as you lift the head.

Now, lift the head just a tiny bit off the floor, helping with the arms, and hold it there. The elbows should be pointing up toward the ceiling. Turn the head left and right, and assist with the arms. As the head turns right, the right elbow moves down toward the floor, and the left elbow moves up away from the floor. The head does not slide in the hands.

Repeat this move for a minute or two, and be sure not to hold your breath. Notice how far the head turns, and how easily. Set the head and arms on the floor and rest briefly.

Lift the head as before, helping with the arms, so that the elbows point to the ceiling. Squeeze the eyes tightly shut, and turn the head left and right as you just did. Notice how the head moves now. Does it turn as far as before? As easily? After a minute, stop squeezing the eyes, and continue to turn the head. How does the head move now? Once again, squeeze the eyes and turn the head. Can you still feel the restriction in the head motion? Stop moving, stretch out, and rest.

Draw up your knees, feet standing, and interlace your fingers behind your head. Helping with the hands, lift the head as far as it will go easily, and then set it back down. Repeat this motion for a minute, and notice how your spine moves in back. Let yourself breathe out easily as you lift the head.

Set your head and arms back down on the floor. Now, squeeze your eyes tightly shut, and then relax them. Squeeze the eyes again, but this time only half as much. Then, squeeze the eyes again, and again reduce the effort by half. Continue to squeeze the eyes, each time reducing the effort by half, until you are making the least perceptible squeezing motion. Repeat this minimal squeezing a number of times, and notice your breathing. Are you holding your breath?

Stop squeezing the eyes. Now, very slowly, begin to lift your head, helping with the hands and arms, as you did before. Do not actually lift the head, just begin to make the movement, so that the pressure of the head and hands against the floor lessens just a little, then cease all effort. Repeat this "move" several times, and notice your eyes. Do you squeeze your eyes as you begin to lift the head?

Continue to start lifting the head, and begin to let go of any squeezing of the eyes. Gradually, increase the lifting of the head, but only as far as you can without squeezing the eyes. Let yourself breathe easily as you do this, and notice the neck, shoulders, and chest. After a few trials, you will probably find that you can lift the head up a several inches without squeezing the eyes. How does it feel to do this? Is it easier to lift the head when you do not squeeze the eyes? Stop moving, stretch out, and rest.

After resting for a minute, roll over to one side, and come up to standing. Did you squeeze your eyes as you stood up? After you stand, check your posture. Are you standing differently? How does your breathing feel? Walk around a little. Is your walk any different?

Over the next few days, think about your eyes from time to time, especially when you feel that you are straining or making an effort to do something. Are you squeezing your eyes? What happens as you become aware of this unneeded effort and stop making it?

10: Standing and shifting 1

For good action, the visual system must be able to locate an object out in space in relation to the body. In order to do this, brain takes in information not only from the eyes, but also from the kinesthetic sense -that is, from the sensations of movement of the body. Thus, in some sense, we see with our whole body, and not just with our eyes. Today we are going to work to improve this function of the visual system.

As usual, remove your glasses or contacts if you wear them, and then do about five minutes of sunning and then another five minutes of palming.

Now, take your yard stick and prop it up so that it is vertical, and so that the top of the stick is just below eye level when you are standing. Arrange the stick and its props so that it is two or three feet in front of a blank wall. Cover your non-dominant eye with the eye patch and stand about five or six feet away from the stick in such a way that a line drawn from your eye through the stick to the wall would meet the wall at a right angle. Make a mental note of just where you are standing, or place some object on the floor to mark your place, so that you can do the whole exercise without changing your position relative to the stick.

Now, take your place facing the stick, and fix your dominant eye on the top of the stick. Holding your eye on the stick, begin to shift your weight toward the side of the eye that is open, and then come back to center. Continue to shift your weight to one side like this, and scan your body with your attention.

Make sure that you continue to face straight toward the stick, and just move your weight from one side to the other. Do not allow your body to turn to the side.

Notice how your weight shifts from the middle, over to one foot, and then back to the middle. Notice your knees. Do they bend at all as you shift your weight? Can you feel your eye ball moving? Does your breathing continue at a normal pace?

After you have done this for one to two minutes, continue to shift your weight as before, but close your eyes, and look at the stick in your imagination. Shift your weight toward the side of the eye that is open, and then back to center, about five or six times, and then stop, and open your eye. Are you really looking at the stick? Repeat this sequence several times, until the position of the imaginary stick coincides with the position of the real stick when you open your eyes.

Now begin to shift your weight to the other side, away from the side of the eye that is open. As before, notice how your body moves, and how the pressure changes on the soles of your feet. Continue to move like this for one or two minutes, keeping your eye on the top comer of the stick.

Continue to shift your weight, but now close your eye, and track the stick in your imagination. As before, go back and forth several times with your eyes closed, and then stop, open your eye, and check to see if the imaginary stick coincides with the real stick. Repeat this several times.

Now combine the two previous movements, and begin to shift your weight left and right, and keep your eye on the stick. Continue for one to two minutes, and notice how your body moves, and how your weight shifts from one foot to the other and back. Can you watch the stick and pay attention to the sensations of movement and weight shifting at the same time? Remember to pay attention to what you can see with your peripheral vision from time to time.

Now continue the previous movement, but close your eyes, and track the stick in your imagination. As before, make five or six moves with your eyes closed, and then stop moving, open your eye, and notice if you are actually looking at the stick. Repeat this sequence five or six times, and then stop.

Take off your eye patch, lie down on the floor, and cover your eyes with the palms of your hands. Compare the left and right visual fields, and notice which one is blacker, and which one extends out to the left and right, and up and down, the most. Move your eyes around a little, and pay attention to the sensations of movement of the eyeball. Which eye moves easier? Which eyeball feels bigger?

Roll to one side, stand up, and put the eye patch on your dominant eye. Return to the place that you marked on the floor, and repeat the previous movements with the non-dominant eye open and watching the stick. Does the non-dominant eye learn as fast as the dominant eye? After you have finished working with the non-dominant eye, take off the eye patch, lie down and palm your eyes.

Stand up, and return to your place on the floor, several feet away from the stick. With both eyes, look at the top of the stick, and begin to shift your weight left and right. Watch the stick, and notice how your weight shifts left and right on the soles of your feet, and how your body moves. Continue to look at the stick, and be aware of how far you can see to the left and right, and up and down.

After two or three minutes of this, continue to move, but close your eyes, and track the stick in your imagination. After shifting your weight several times with your eyes closed, stop, open your eyes, and note if you are really looking at the stick. Repeat this sequence several times, until the position of the imaginary stick and the position of the real stick coincide.

Now, shift your weight from left to right a few times with your eyes closed, and then stop moving with your weight in the middle. Keeping your eyes closed, step forward and grab the stick.

Make a single grab and stop, and then open your eyes. If you don't get the stick on your first try, go back to your place on the floor, shift your weight left and right with your eyes open and then closed, and then make another grab at the stick. Be sure to start from the same place on the floor each time.

As you go for the stick, do not make any special effort to hit it. Have the attitude that you would have if your eyes were open. If you proceed in this way, you will find that it is easy to grab the stick.

After you have grabbed the stick several times, return to your place and shift your weight left and right a few times, with your eyes open and then closed. Is there any change in your internal representation of the stick -that is, does the imaginary stick that you see with your eyes closed seem different in any way?

Lie down on the floor and palm your eyes for several minutes, then stand up and look around. How does the world look?

The next time that you do this exercise, stand a little further away from the stick, and at the end, try to grab the stick from this increased distance. How far away can you start and still get the stick?

11: Standing and shifting 2

Today we are going to work with one of the most basic operations of the visual system. When we look at two objects, we have to be able to see which is closer, and which is farther away, and how the movements of our body will affect the spatial relationships between the eyes and the objects. Having a proper internal representation of this spatial relationship will improve action.

To begin, remove your glasses or contacts if you wear them, and then do about five minutes of sunning, and then another five minutes of palming.

Now, take your yard stick and prop it up just as you did in the previous chapter, so that it is vertical, and the top is slightly below eye level. The stick should be two or three feet in front of a blank wall. Take a second stick, and place it about two feet further away from the wall than the first stick. This second stick should also be vertical, and the top should be just below eye level. Arrange the two sticks so that a line drawn through the sticks would meet the wall at a right angle.

Cover your non-dominant eye with the eye patch, and stand about five to seven feet away from the second stick. Adjust your position so that your eye sights over the near stick to the far one. In this position, the near stick covers most of the far stick, but you should be able to see the very top of the far stick. Mark your place on the floor so that you can do the whole exercise at a constant distance from the two sticks.

As you stand there facing the sticks, begin to shift your weight toward the eye that is open, and then back toward the middle. Continue to do this, and keep your eye focused on the top of the near stick. Notice how your weight shifts onto one foot, and then back to the middle, and how your body moves. As you shift your weight to one side, notice how the far stick appears to move out to the same side away from the near stick. Then, as you shift your weight back toward the middle, the far stick moves back in line with the near stick. Repeat this motion for about two minutes, letting yourself breathe easily.

Continue to move in this way, close your eyes, and see the two sticks in your imagination. Shift your weight several times with your eyes closed, and notice if the imaginary sticks seem to move in the same way as the real sticks. Then, open your eyes and observe the real sticks. Do the imaginary sticks and the real sticks actually move in the same way? Repeat this sequence several times, following the imaginary sticks with your eyes closed, and then opening your eyes and comparing your imaginary, internal representation of the sticks, with the real sticks.

Close your eyes, and shift your weight to the side and back to the middle several times, while following the imaginary sticks with your mind's eye. Stop moving when the two imaginary sticks are lined up. Open your eye. Are the sticks really lined up? Repeat this several times until you can line the sticks up with your eyes closed. Does it help to pay attention to the sensation of pressure on the bottoms of your feet as you do this? Stop moving and rest for a minute.

Stand as before, so that the two sticks appear to be lined up with your eye. Now begin to shift your weight away from the eye that is open, and then back toward the middle. Continue to do this and keep your eye fixed on the near stick. Notice how the far stick appears to move out to the side from behind the near stick, in the direction in which you are shifting your weight. As you move, let yourself breathe easily, and be aware of the sensations of motion in your body, and the shift of weight on the sales of your feet. Repeat this movement for about two minutes.

Now, continue to move, but close your eyes, and watch the two sticks in your imagination. Does the far stick appear to move out to the side in the same direction in which you are shifting your weight? Make several shifts with your eyes open, and then several with your eyes closed, then open, and so on.

Continue to shift your weight with your eyes closed, and stop when you "see" that the two imaginary sticks are lined up. Open your eyes. Are the two sticks actually lined up with your eye? Repeat this several times, and then stop and rest for a minute.

Stand as before, and now combine the two previous movements by shifting your weight from left to right and back. Keep your eye focused on the top of the near stick, and observe how the far stick appears to move out to the side in the direction in which you shift your weight. Notice your breathing, and how your weight shifts from one side to the other on the soles of your feet.

After about two minutes of this, close your eyes and continue the movement, following the sticks in your imagination. Can you get the sense that the two sticks are out in front of you somewhere, separated by a certain distance, and that this particular configuration of the two sticks and your eye are the cause of the far stick moving out to the side as you shift your weight?

Shift a few times with your eyes closed, and then a few more times with your eyes open, and then closed, and so on. As you do this notice how the position of the internal, imaginary sticks, begins to match the position of the real sticks.

With your eyes closed, stop with the imaginary sticks lined up. Open your eyes. Are the two sticks really lined up? Repeat this several times. Stop and rest for a minute, but do not remove the eye patch.

Stand as before, with the two sticks lined up with your eye. Direct your eye to the top of the far stick, and begin to shift your weight toward the eye that is open. Continue to do this, and keep your eye focused on the top of the far stick. Notice how your weight shifts onto one foot, and then back to the middle, and how your body moves. As you shift your weight to one side, notice how the near stick appears to move out to the opposite side away from the far stick. Then, as you shift your weight back toward the middle, the near stick moves back in line with the far stick. Repeat this motion for about two minutes, letting yourself breathe easily.

Continue to move in this way, close your eyes, and see the two sticks in your imagination. Shift your weight several times with your eyes closed, and notice if the imaginary sticks seem to move in the same way as the real sticks. Then, open your eyes and observe the real sticks. Do the imaginary sticks and the real sticks actually move in the same way? Repeat this sequence several times, following the imaginary sticks with your eyes closed, and then opening your eyes and comparing your imaginary, internal representation of the sticks, with the real sticks.

Close your eyes, and shift your weight to the side and back to the middle several times, while following the imaginary sticks with your mind's eye. Stop moving when the two imaginary sticks are lined up. Open your eye. Are the sticks really lined up? Repeat this several times until you can line the sticks up with your eyes closed. Does it help to pay attention to the sensation of pressure on the bottoms of your feet as you do this? Stop moving and rest for a minute.

Stand as before, so that the two sticks appear to be lined up with your eye. Now begin to shift your weight away from the eye that is open, and then back toward the middle. Continue to do this and keep your eye fixed on the far stick. Notice how the near stick appears to move out to the side from the front of the far stick, in the opposite direction in which you are shifting your weight. As you move, let yourself breathe easily, and be aware of the sensations of motion in your body, and of the shift of weight on the soles of your feet. Repeat this movement for about two minutes.

Now, continue to move, but close your eyes, and watch the two sticks in your imagination. Does the near stick appear to move out to the side in the opposite direction to which you are shifting your weight? Make several shifts with your eyes open, and then several with your eyes closed, then open, and so on.

Continue to shift your weight with your eyes closed, and stop when you "see" that the two imaginary sticks are lined up. Open your eyes. Are the two sticks actually lined up with your eye? Repeat this several times, and then stop and rest for a minute.

Stand as before, and now combine the two previous movements by shifting your weight from left to right and back. Keep your eye focused on the top of the far stick, and observe how the near stick appears to move out to the side in the direction opposite to which you shift your weight... Notice your breathing, and how your weight shifts from one side to the other on the soles of your feet.

After about t wo minutes of this, close your eyes and continue the movement, following the sticks in your imagination. Can you get the sense that the two stick are out in front of you somewhere, separated by a certain distance, and that this particular configuration of the two sticks and your eye are the cause of the near stick moving out to the side as you shift your weight?

Shift a few times with your eyes closed, and then a few more times with your eyes open, and then closed, and so on. As you do this notice how the internal, imaginary sticks, begin to match the real sticks.

With your eyes closed, stop with the imaginary sticks lined up. Open your eyes. Are the two sticks really lined up? Repeat this several times. Stop and rest for a minute, but do not remove the eye patch.

Once again, stand so that the two sticks are lined up with your eye. Begin to shift your weight left and right. Shift your weight several times with your eye directed to the top of the far stick, and notice how the near stick appears to move, and then continue to shift your weight while you look at the top of the near stick, and notice how the far stick appears to move. Move slowly, pay attention to the sensations of movement in your body, and to the shift of pressure on the bottoms of your feet, and allow yourself to breathe easily. Go back and forth between the two sticks several times, and open your peripheral vision from time to time so that you are aware of your whole visual field.

Continue to shift your weight left and right, and close your eyes.· now "look" at either the far or the near stick in your imagination, and notice how the other stick moves. With your eyes closed, "look" at one stick, then the other, and so on. Do the imaginary sticks move in the same way as the real ones? That is, when you are "looking" at the near stick in your imagination, does the far stick appear to move in the same direction that you shift your weight, and when you are "looking" at the far stick, does the near stick appear to move in the opposite direction to the shift of weight? Open your eyes and check the movements of the real sticks if you have any questions about how the sticks move. Stop moving, take off the eye patch, and lie down and palm your eyes.

As you lie there, compare the blackness of the left and right visual fields. Which is blacker? Move your eyes around a little. Which eye moves more easily? Sit up, open your eyes, and look around. Can you detect a difference between the vision of the two eyes?

Stand up, return to your place on the floor, and place the eye patch over your dominant eye. Repeat the entire exercise with the non-dominant eye. Do you find it less easy to visualize (that is, with your eyes closed) the relative movements of the two sticks with your non-dominant eye? If so, what can this tell you about the relationship between the mental qualities of perception, which we usually call imagination or visualization, and the physical qualities, such as the shape of the eyeball, and the flexibility of the lens and the muscles around the eyes?

When you are finished, go outside where you can see some trees, and shift your weight left and right while looking at the trunks and limbs. Notice how the trees appear to move in the same way as the sticks. Walk around while looking at the trees. What do you see?

Notes

12: V - X - A exercise

In all of the previous exercises we have worked mainly with the eyes one at a time, but of course, in our day to day life, we use the eyes together. In this lesson, we are going to begin to work with both eyes at once, and to improve the way in which the eyes work together.

As usual, remove glasses or contacts if you wear them, and begin with about five minutes of sunning and then another five minutes of palming.

Now uncover your eyes, stand up, and arrange a straight backed, armless chair so that the back of the chair faces a blank section of wall. The chair should be about five to seven feet away from the wall. Take your stick and place two different colored pushpins in the long narrow side. Put one pin at one end of the stick, and one in the middle. Sit down on the chair so that you straddle the back, and face the wall. Cover your non-dominant eye with the eye patch. As you do the exercise, rest your elbows on the on the back of the chair to give your arms support. Use a pad on the chair back to raise the support up far enough so that you do not have to slump to rest your elbows.

Now hold the stick up so that the end without a pin is touching your nose. The stick should be horizontal, and pointing straight out in front, toward the wall, and the pushpins should be on the top edge of the stick. As you look out along the stick with one eye, you see the long wide side of the stick, and the pushpins, which are stuck in the long narrow side of the stick.

Now look at the wall straight out in front, then look at the far pushpin, then sweep your eye slowly down the stick to the near pushpin, and then continue on and sweep your eye on down the stick to your nose. Then, reverse the motion, letting your eye move out along the stick to the near push-pin, then on out to the far one, and then on out to the wall. Continue to do this for one to two minutes, and let yourself breathe easily, and from time to time be aware of all that you can see with your peripheral vision.

Continue to sweep your eye in and out like this, but have your eyes closed. Make a few sweeps with your eyes closed, then a few more with your eyes open, then closed, and so on. Set the stick down and rest in the chair briefly.

Bring the stick back to the initial position, with one end touching the nose, and the stick held horizontally straight out in front, as before. Move the far end of the stick in the direction of the eye that is open about three or four inches. The near end of the stick is still touching the tip of the nose. Holding the stick still, begin to sweep the eye in and out along the stick as you did before. Let the eye sweep slowly along the stick and out to the wall and back, and pause at each of the pins. Let yourself breathe easily, and notice what you can see with your peripheral vision. Continue to do this for one to two minutes, and then continue the motion, but with your eyes closed. Make a few sweeps with your eyes closed, then open, then closed, and so on. Set the stick down and rest in the chair.

Pick up the stick and hold it straight out in front horizontally, as before. Pivoting the stick about the nose, move the far end of the stick a little to the side, away from the eye that is open. Move the stick until the two pins appear to be lined up, so that the near pin covers the far one, then move the far end of the stick back toward the center line of the body a tiny fraction of an inch so that you can see both pins.

As before, look at the wall in front of the stick, then at the far pushpin, then sweep your eye in along the stick to the near pushpin, and then on in to your nose, then reverse the movement and go out along the stick until you get to the wall. Repeat for one to two minutes, and then continue with your eyes closed. Go in and out several times with the eyes closed, then a few more times with the eyes open, then closed, and so on.

Stop moving, take off the patch, lie down and palm your eyes. Compare the sensations of the left and right visual fields. Move the eyes about some. Which eye moves easier? Open your eyes, stand up, and look around. Which eye sees more clearly?

Go back to the chair and cover your dominant eye with the patch. Repeat the previous movements with the non-dominant eye. Begin with the stick straight out in front, then work with the far end of the stick over to the side of the eye that is open, and then work with the far end of the stick over to the side of the eye that is covered, so that the two pins appear to be lined up. Remember to breathe as you move, and to notice what you can see with your peripheral vision. Remove the patch, and lie down and palm your eyes for a few minutes when you are finished.

Go back to the chair and hold the stick as before, with one end touching the nose, and the stick horizontal and straight out in front. There is a pushpin in the far end of the stick, and one in the middle. You are not wearing the eye patch.

Look at the near pin, and notice that you see two of the far pins. Then, look at the far pin, and notice that you see two of the near pins. Go back and forth between the far pin and the near pin a number of times until this becomes clear. Then look at the wall, straight out in front. Now you will see two of each pin, a total of four. Look at the near end of the stick, and you will again see four pins. Spend a few minutes exploring these sensations, letting your eyes sweep in and out along the stick.

Notice that you see two sticks as you do this. When you look at the near end of the stick, the two sticks meet at your nose and appear to form a letter v. When you look at the near pushpin, in the middle of the stick, the two sticks appear to cross in the middle and form a letter x. Then, when you look at the far pushpin, the two sticks appear to meet at the far end, and look like a letter a without the cross piece. This gives the name v-x-a to this exercise.

Rest briefly, then hold the stick up again. Look at the far pin. Begin to wave the stick slowly left and right, pivoting about the nose, and move the stick far enough to each side so that the near pin hides the far pin. Let yourself breathe easily, and be aware of your peripheral vision. Do you move an equal amount to each side to line up the pins on that side?

Rest briefly, then hold the stick as before. Look at the far pin, and swing the stick over to one side, pivoting about the nose, until one of the near pins covers the far one.

Hold the stick in this position, and look at the near pin, then sweep your eyes out along the stick and look at the far pin, then look at the near pin, and so on. Remember to breathe, and to pay attention to your peripheral vision as you do this.

Move the stick over to the other side and repeat the previous movement, sweeping your eyes in and out along the stick. Stop and rest briefly.

Bring the stick back up to your face, straight out in front. Move the near end of the stick an inch away from your nose. Holding the stick still, turn your head left and right a little so that your nose moves to each side about one inch. Continue to turn your head, and sweep your eyes in and out along the stick. Look at the wall, then at the far pin, then at the near pin, then at the close end of the stick, then at the near pin, and so on. Repeat for a minute, and remember to breathe, and to be aware of your peripheral vision. Stop moving, lie down, and palm your eyes for a few minutes.

Uncover your eyes, stand up, and look around. Go outside and look. Does your sense of the three dimensionality of the world seem enhanced?

Notes

13: Convergence card

In chapter eight, we worked with convergence, or the ability of both eyes to focus on a single point. In this chapter, we are going to work with convergence in a different way. By using a target, called a convergence card, in a certain way, we can present a different image to each eye in such a way that the eyes fuse the two images to form one image, and you will see a figure that does not actually exist.

As usual, remove glasses or contacts if you wear them, and then do about five minutes of sunning, and then another five minutes of palming.

Take an ordinary business card, and copy the design shown at the end of the introduction onto the blank side of the card. Be certain that the two circles are positioned in an exactly symmetrical fashion about the vertical center line of the card, so that the images will fuse properly. Cut out the crosshatched section of the card and adjust the width so that it just fits over the yardstick. Cut the card so that it grabs onto the stick firmly, without deforming the card.

Take your yardstick, and remove any pushpins that you have in it. Put the convergence card on the stick, about in the middle, so that the card is perpendicular to the four long edges of the stick. Arrange your chair facing away from a section of blank wall, about six or eight feet away. Place the eye patch over the non-dominant eye and sit straddling the chair, facing the wall. Use the back of the chair for an arm rest if you wish.

Hold the stick up horizontally, and straight out in front, so that one end touches the bridge of the nose, just between the eyes. Look out along the stick so that you see the circle on one side of the card with the eye that is open. The stick blocks the other circle from the view of the uncovered eye.

Sweep your eye in and out along the stick a few times, and notice exactly what you see. Let yourself breathe easily, and notice what you can see with your peripheral vision. Move the card in closer and sweep your eye in and out along the stick a few times, and then move the card out near the end of the stick and sweep your eye in and out. After about five minutes of this, switch the patch over to the dominant eye, and go through this whole procedure again with the non-dominant eye. When you are finished, remove the eye patch and lie down and palm your eyes.

As you lie there, remember what you saw with each eye as you looked out along the stick. With each eye, you saw a circle, just to the side of the stick. One circle had a horizontal diameter drawn in it, and the other had a vertical diameter. When the right eye was open, the circle was to the right of the stick. When the left eye was open, the circle was to the left of the stick.

In your mind's eye, put the right and left images together, as if both eyes were uncovered. What do you "see?"

Go back to your chair and sit as before. Hold the stick horizontally straight out in front, with one end touching the bridge of the nose, just between the eyes. Both eyes are uncovered. The convergence card should be about in the middle of the stick, with the circles facing you.

Sweep your eyes in and out along the stick, slowly, and at a certain point you will see the two circles fuse into one circle, with a cross in the middle. The circle appears to be between two sticks. If you do not get this right away, experiment with moving the card further away from your eyes, or closer to them.

When you get the two circles to fuse, move your eyes around the circle in one direction, and then the other, and up and down and left and right across the two arms of the cross. Do both arms of the cross (that is, the left eye and the right eye images) appear equally clear?

Move the end of the stick away from your face about an inch, and slowly turn your head left and right a little. The stick remains still. Your nose will move about a half inch to each side.

Can you maintain the illusion of a single circle with a cross in the middle as you move your head? Try nodding your head up and down, and then move your nose in clockwise and counter clockwise circles as you look at the circle with the cross. Let yourself breathe easily as you move your head. Move the card a little closer, and then a little further away, and experiment with fusing the circles. Is there a distance where it is particularly easy for you to do this? Is there a distance where it is particularly difficult?

Lie down and palm your eyes some more. Once again try to fuse the circles in your imagination. Is it· easier now?

After a few minutes of palming, open your eyes, stand up, and look around. How does the world look to you?

Other Titles by Jack Heggie
from *Feldenkrais* Resources

Running With the Whole Body, Jack Heggie

A *Feldenkrais* perspective on running including eleven *Awareness Through Movement* lessons. Each exercise is illustrated with photographs and case studies.
Softbound book
Item # 1172

Total Body Golf, Jack Heggie

Jack Heggie developed many ATM lessons for the particular needs of athletes. Each lesson in this set is oriented to specific functional abilities which are required for an outstanding golf swing. Three CDs include 7 ATM lessons and an introduction.
3 CD set
Item # 1498

Total Body Vision, Jack Heggie

Through a series of eleven original lessons on six CD's and drawing on the *Feldenkrais Method* and the work of William Bates, M.D., Jack Heggie developed a powerful series of exercises for improving the overall quality of your vision, posture, and movement. The lessons will facilitate eye-hand and eye-foot coordination, color and depth perception, and create greater ease in discerning texture and fine detail
6 CD set
Item # 1499

Please visit our website to order and view a large selection of books, DVDs and audio CDs on the *Feldenkrais* Method®.
www.feldenkraisresources.com
Toll Free: 800-756-1907

Notes

Notes

Notes

Notes

Made in the USA
San Bernardino, CA
20 November 2015